*Understanding*

# COMPLEMENTARY MEDICINE

Dr George T Lewith


| KENT LIBRARIES AND ARCHIVES | |
|---|---|
| C152872768 | |
| Bertrams | 03.07.06 |
| | £3.50 |
| | |


Publi

in as

## IMPORTANT NOTICE

This book is intended not as a substitute for personal medical advice but as a supplement to that advice for the patient who wishes to understand more about his/her condition.

Before taking any form of treatment YOU SHOULD ALWAYS CONSULT YOUR MEDICAL PRACTITIONER.

In particular (without limit) you should note that advances in medical science occur rapidly and some of the information about drugs and treatment contained in this booklet may very soon be out of date.

All rights reserved. No part of this publication may be reproduced, or stored in a retrieval system, or transmitted, in any form or by any means, electronic, mechanical, photocopying, recording and/or otherwise, without the prior written permission of the publishers. The right of Dr George T Lewith to be identified as the author of this work has been asserted in accordance with the Copyright, Designs and Patents Act 1988, Sections 77 and 78.

© Family Doctor Publications 2002, 2004
Updated 2004

Family Doctor Publications, PO Box 4664, Poole, Dorset BH15 1NN

**Medical Editor:** Dr Tony Smith
**Consultant Editors:** Victoria Goldman, Mary Fox, Chris McLaughlin
**Cover Artist:** Dave Eastbury
**Medical Artist:** Peter Cox Associates
**Design:** Peter Powell Origination & Print Limited
**Printing:** Nuffield Press, Abingdon, using acid-free paper

**ISBN: 1 903474 05 1**

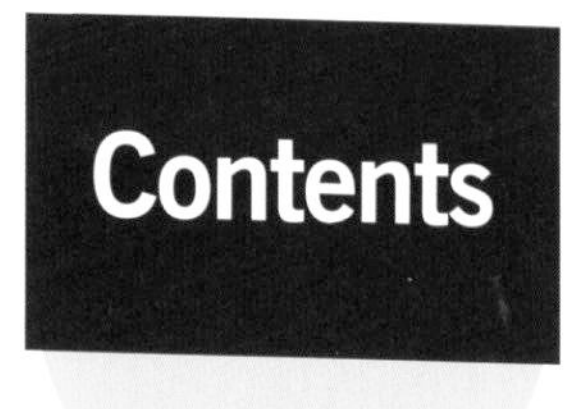

# Contents

# Introduction

Complementary medicine is a term that covers many unrelated therapies. However, many people now prefer to use the term 'complementary and alternative medicine' (CAM) instead and this will be used, where appropriate, throughout this book.

In the late 1950s and early 1960s, treatments such as acupuncture were considered to be fringe medicine. Then, in the 1970s and early 1980s, they began to be called 'alternative' because they were thought to represent an alternative to conventional medicine.

During the late 1980s and 1990s, the term changed to 'complementary' as doctors and 'alternative' therapists began working together, using treatments to complement conventional medical care. In some instances, CAM treatments have now been integrated into conventional medicine – for example, many physiotherapists use acupuncture on their patients.

When complementary medicine is used as part of a complete package of treatment including conventional medicine, the term 'integrated medicine' is used – for example, the increasing use of homeopathy by GPs as a part of their ordinary medical practice once a clear conventional diagnosis has been made. In other words, such doctors are integrating the CAM therapy into their conventional care.

The changes in terminology show how much attitudes have changed over the last 40 years – among both the public and the medical profession. From thinking of CAM therapies as quackery in the 1950s and 1960s, we now regard them as techniques that may be used in NHS hospitals and health centres.

The underlying reason for this change is unclear, but it is probably partly because patients and doctors now recognise that there are benefits to be derived from CAM and partly because of changes in the attitudes of doctors to CAM.

How can we define CAM? One way is 'therapies that are alien to the dominant healthcare system of a specific country'. For example, acupuncture and herbal medicine are considered to be conventional in China, but unconventional in the USA and UK. Another definition is 'techniques that are not taught in medical school'. However, healthcare systems do change over time and many UK medical schools now offer CAM familiarisation courses.

There is a whole range of complementary therapies and the table represents a broad, but far from comprehensive, list. A number of these therapies are discussed in more detail in this book.

## Are CAM therapies related?

Some therapies are related to one another; acupuncture, acupressure, reiki, shiatsu and traditional Chinese herbal remedies are all used in accordance with traditional Chinese medical concepts. However, most CAM therapies are an unrelated mixture of treatments with entirely different histories, philosophies and uses. Ayurveda (a comprehensive Indian traditional medical approach to illness) involves diet, yoga, massage and herbal remedies and, although many of the Ayurvedic herbal remedies are similar to those used by the Chinese, there are also significant differences.

Both systems, Indian and Chinese, have evolved over the last 2,000 years into complete medical approaches that involve diagnosis and treatment. Homeopathy, on the other hand, is entirely unrelated to any other form of CAM and was developed 200 years ago in Germany. There are many manual therapies, such as osteopathy, chiropractic, massage and the Alexander technique, that are designed to affect the body through various forms of touching or manipulation.

As most CAM treatments are entirely unrelated, in many instances the therapy chosen is dependent on the disorder and the knowledge and beliefs of the patient, doctor and CAM practitioner.

## Is CAM safe and natural?

Some patients are made ill by conventional medicine. Estimates suggest that complications occur in

## COMMON COMPLEMENTARY THERAPIES

**Therapies that have a connection with traditional Chinese medicine**

Acupressure
Acupuncture
Herbal medicine
Reiki
Shiatsu

**Therapies that have a connection with Ayurvedic (traditional Hindu) medicine**

Aromatherapy
Herbal medicine
Yoga

**Massage and manipulative-based therapies**

Chiropractic
Cranial osteopathy
Massage
Osteopathy
Reflexology

**Mind–body therapies**

Autogenic training
Biofeedback
Healing
Hypnosis
Meditation
Relaxation and visualisation
Therapeutic touch

**Naturopathy-related therapies**

Environmental medicine
Naturopathy
Nutritional medicine

**Unique therapies**

Homeopathy

as many as five per cent of operations, and many people taking long-term conventional medication experience some side effects. However, conventional drugs are often given to very sick, frail, old people who are more likely to have an adverse reaction.

The media sometimes seem to imply that many complementary therapies have magical properties and, unlike conventional medicines, could not possibly harm you. It is important to remember that 'natural' does not always mean safe. Herbal and nutritional products produced in environments where their quality of manufacture is uncontrolled may be dangerously contaminated and far from safe.

In spite of these concerns, CAM treatments seem, on the whole, to be far less likely than conventional medicines to have serious side effects or complications. However, we need to know more about the safety of CAM treatments and the possibility of interactions with conventional medicines. If you are taking a herbal, homeopathic or nutritional product, you must tell your GP so that any adverse reaction to a conventional medicine or any interaction with your prescribed remedies can be identified.

Many CAM therapists claim to be holistic – that is, treating the whole person not just a specific problem. This might suggest that conventional medicine is not 'whole person' medicine. In fact, good conventional medicine does take into account the whole person, and some CAM therapies themselves are very narrow and specialised.

An important potential danger with CAM is that a patient may not receive appropriate conventional treatment because the non-medically qualified CAM practitioner is unable to make a proper medical diagnosis. As a result of this, the patient is given inadequate and potentially dangerous advice and may miss out on the best conventional treatments available. Although this may have happened in some instances, specific cases of patients receiving inappropriate treatment have rarely been reported in the medical literature. In fact, most CAM therapists are now over-cautious and are more likely to over-refer you to your GP than under-refer you if they are in any doubt.

If you follow the guidelines and advice about seeking CAM treatment given in the chapter 'Who provides complementary therapies?' (page 91), then this should mean that your GP is fully informed about your treatment and that it is both appropriate for you and based on a clear and safe diagnosis.

## What do CAM therapies share?

Many CAM therapies share an unscientific, unproven and possibly unprovable belief that a vital force or vital energy is present in living organisms. This belief underpins many of the CAM approaches to illness, and it is the manipulation of this vital energy that is the main aim of some therapies.

With this approach, chronic illness is thought to be caused by a prolonged disturbance in the body's energy. This energetic disturbance ultimately leads to disease that can be seen and described in conventional medical terms. Treatment is therefore designed to rebalance the person's vital energy.

In some therapies, such as osteopathy and chiropractic, the current teaching and practice has completely distanced itself from these unproven assumptions about vital force. Some CAM therapists believe that illness provides an opportunity for the person to change, suggesting that illness has a deeper meaning.

With almost all CAM therapies, the person receiving treatment may find their symptoms or illness is aggravated as part of the healing process. The original condition may become temporarily worse, or the symptoms may revert to those that were apparent when the illness began. These changes are claimed to support the idea of a natural healing process that is stimulated by a particular therapy, although there is no scientific basis for this.

Many CAM therapies, and the individual treatments that are prescribed within each of them, are very 'empirical' – this means that they are based on experience of success rather than an understanding of theory. In conventional medicine, people like to think that they understand much more about the treatments they practise, and indeed they often do, yet even conventional doctors use treatments that might be considered empirical.

## Does CAM work?

More is known about the clinical effectiveness of CAM now than 10 or 15 years ago. Some particular therapies are known to be safe and effective in certain conditions, but lack of understanding about the specific effects of CAM is still enormous.

For most CAM therapies, we do not understand a great deal about the mechanism of how a therapy works and indeed whether it works better than a placebo (inactive substance used in control trials to establish the specific effectiveness of a treatment). The main reason for this is that not much research has been published on the effectiveness of CAM.

CAM attracts less than one per cent of the research money that goes into conventional medicine, so it is not surprising that not enough is known about these therapies. This lack of information is sometimes seen as a good reason for doctors not recommending CAM. As there is insufficient research information, we can't predict how well or badly a particular treatment may work for an individual or for a particular condition.

It may seem that conventional medicine uses treatments only if they are supported by clinical evidence. In general practice and some hospital medicine, this is not always the case. A lot of treatments your GP prescribes have limited evidence to support them, yet they are very effective.

## Do I need to believe in complementary medicine for it to work?

There have been some suggestions that the only reason that CAM works is because people believe in it. On the few occasions that this assumption has been exposed to proper scrutiny, it has been found that the outcome of treatment is not dependent on whether you believe it is going to work for you.

However, people seeking CAM are more likely to be well-informed about health in general and CAM in particular, and have a greater desire to take control of the factors that affect their health and well-being, such as diet and exercise.

## Can complementary medicine be used with conventional medicine?

In spite of the lack of scientific evidence, many people are convinced that CAM may offer approaches to their illness that are relatively safe and potentially effective. Many people are beginning to ask their GPs whether using a complementary therapy can be effective for them. Most people do not wish to reject conventional medicine, but use it in a more considered way while embracing a complementary approach if it is safe and reasonable to do so.

Patients are therefore making their medical practitioners consider whether CAM can be safely integrated into the management of their illness. For example, a patient with arthritis may wish to use acupuncture or a glucosamine supplement to manage pain rather than conventional medication such as anti-inflammatories, while taking a powerful medication to suppress the aggressive inflammation occurring in their joints.

A recent report from the British Medical Association wholly endorsed the use of acupuncture in pain – an unusual event as far as CAM is concerned. CAM should not be seen as a complete alternative to the management of most illnesses, although undoubtedly in some cases (such as the use of manipulative techniques for acute back pain) it is a safe and effective alternative to visiting your GP.

## Which therapies are most popular?

There have been a number of surveys assessing the most popular therapies in the UK. They show that acupuncture, chiropractic, osteopathy, herbal medicine, homeopathy and, in one survey, faith healing are the most frequently sought CAM treatments. The situation is similar in Europe and the USA.

## Who uses CAM?

Most CAM in the UK is paid for privately, although the NHS does provide some. This means that it is mostly used by those who can afford it. In general, those using complementary medicine are better educated, and 60 per cent are female. Most are in their middle years (between the ages of 40 and 60).

Ethnic communities, particularly Indian and Chinese, tend to use techniques that may be considered complementary in this country but traditional in their country of origin. Unfortunately, there is not much information in the UK on how ethnic groups use CAM. In the USA, it is known that ethnic groups tend to use traditional remedies such as herbs before going to their family physician.

## What gets treated?

Most people seek CAM when they have long-term chronic problems that are poorly managed by conventional medicine, usually with their muscles, bones and joints. They are most likely to seek help for these problems from qualified manipulators such as osteopaths and chiropractors. Sometimes the problems cannot be diagnosed by conventional medical techniques – for example, a general feeling of unwellness or inappropriate exhaustion – or sometimes they can only be managed and not cured, like arthritis.

More and more people are seeing complementary practitioners so that they can maintain their health and develop their own culture of wellness and balance, rather than waiting for illness to strike unexpectedly. As yet there is no clinical evidence for the success of this approach.

## KEY POINTS

- ✓ Complementary and alternative medicine (CAM) covers a range of therapies, some of which are related
- ✓ CAM treatments are generally safe
- ✓ More research is needed for understanding of when and how to use CAM therapies
- ✓ Most CAM therapies have belief in 'vital energy' as the basis for well-being
- ✓ Ideally, CAM should be integrated with conventional medical care

# CAM versus conventional medicine

Ultimately, medicine that has been proved to be both safe and effective is the kind of medicine that all doctors would like to practise, and indeed all patients would like to receive. This must include not only whether the therapies work, but also the risks and benefits of a particular treatment. For instance, the risk of using acupuncture to help back pain is far smaller than the risk of an operation on the back.

In good-quality integrated medicine, the doctor considers safe, low-risk options first, provided that there is some evidence that they work. For procedures that are more invasive and have greater risk, the evidence for their effectiveness would have to be stronger before they are recommended.

Complementary alternative medicine (CAM) largely involves low-tech and safe treatments, so the medical profession has become increasingly more sympathetic towards it. This is particularly so for chronic conditions or situations in which conventional medicine either carries a high risk or has little to offer.

## A different view of illness

Many CAM therapies embrace the view that an illness starts off as a sustained imbalance in the patient's vital energy. They may be suffering from symptoms of irritable bowel syndrome (tummy pain, abdominal distension, flatulence and diarrhoea), possibly because of stress or because their digestive system does not tolerate a particular food.

If these symptoms persist or come on very rapidly, they may be a sign of a more serious illness that may need detailed investigation. In conventional medicine, the GP may not consider the problem to be serious until more symptoms, such as bleeding or weight loss, occur. However, in most complementary medical treatments, this may be less important as the practitioner may be trying to treat the energy imbalance and symptoms first, and thereby return the patient to a sense of well-being.

In general, the CAM practitioner will try to understand the cause of the illness rather than just treat the symptoms. Irritable bowel syndrome may respond to a specific diet or some form of relaxation technique if food intolerance or stress is the main trigger, and this may avoid the long-term use of conventional medical treatments.

The disadvantage of this view of illness is that the CAM practitioner may not be aware of the development of a serious problem, such as cancer, and therefore may not give the best advice. It is therefore vital that you have a proper medical diagnosis before seeking CAM treatment so that as much information as possible is available before treatment starts.

## The value of modern medicine

The advances made in modern medicine over the last 50 years have been of enormous value in both acute (rapid onset) and chronic (long-lasting) illness. Modern management of heart attacks has vastly improved life expectancy, and the use of hip replacements has been of huge benefit for people with arthritis in this joint.

Unfortunately, a few people fail to recognise this and consider that various CAM therapies have the potential to replace conventional medicine in life-threatening conditions. This is a false assumption and one that may lead to inappropriate and unsafe treatment.

## An individualised approach

Conventional medicine is very firmly based on thinking about how a particular illness, or a particular intervention, may affect patients in general. For instance, you may be told that the chances of success from a particular procedure are 50 or 80 per cent. A particular diagnosis will have several possible treatments, each with their own risks and probabilities of success.

The aim in CAM treatment is to individualise the approach. For example, a patient with a headache consulting a homeopath may be prescribed any one of 30 or 40 remedies, depending on their general constitution and their detailed symptoms. To arrive at a prescription, the homeopath spends time with the patient finding out about the individual's symptoms in great detail.

This personalised approach is found in many CAM therapies and may contribute to patient satisfaction.

## Holism?

Holism is the name given to the treatment of the 'whole person'. Both conventional medicine and CAM try to use a holistic approach.

If you have a persistent headache, your GP will consider whether it is triggered by a small tumour or, far more likely, by stress, sinusitis or difficulties with your neck. By looking at both physical and psychological options, the GP is being holistic – taking into account the whole person and their social and emotional environment.

Most CAM approaches are holistic but some can be very specialist and focused. For example, if you approached a chiropractor with a headache, he or she might manipulate only your neck, which in many ways would be a very specialist and non-holistic approach.

The claim therefore that complementary medicine is the same as holism is not necessarily true but, by and large, the example previously given of the homeopathic approach to treating a headache is far more common than the example of chiropractic treatment directed at the neck.

## Chronic conditions

Most people seeking help from CAM do so because they have chronic conditions. These conditions are often not in themselves life threatening. They are frequently managed conventionally with long-term medication that may result, over a period of years, in some form of adverse reaction, as can happen with drugs used for arthritis.

People with these conditions may be drawn to CAM partly because such treatments generally have a low risk of serious adverse effects. The limited evidence available suggests that the CAM treatments in themselves rarely cure the illness, but may help the patient cope with it more easily and, therefore, may improve his or her quality of life.

Treatments with conventional medicine are often dramatic and immediate – for example, treating acute arthritis with conventional drugs can result in remarkable improvement over a period of a week or two. This almost never occurs in complementary medicine – the effects of a treatment are usually slow to appear. It may take some months before a real and consistent benefit emerges.

You should have a realistic expectation of what CAM may achieve for you. If you have long-term arthritis and take a homeopathic or herbal remedy and after four to six months of treatment there is no obvious benefit, you should consider whether the approach you are using has any value. CAM treatments may take a long time to work, but this should not be an excuse for your practitioner to ask you to visit every month or two for ever!

## TIME AND MONEY

In this country, most complementary medicine is within the private sector and only a small proportion of it is covered by medical insurance. This means that most people visiting a complementary therapist pay for their consultation themselves. They also will usually have more time spent with them than if they saw their GP.

These two factors – payment and length of consultation – may contribute to the success of CAM. It has been suggested that CAM may not have a specific therapeutic benefit but that the environment in which it is practised and the payment involved are really what provides the clinical effect. Researchers describe this as a non-specific, or placebo, effect, which is a general effect not related to treatment. However, the evidence that time and money are significant factors in the effectiveness of complementary medicine is not available, although these suggestions are not unreasonable.

## AM I TREATED AS AN EQUAL BY THE CAM PRACTITIONER?

Patients who seek CAM feel that the whole consultation process is much more equal and therefore more satisfying than consultation with a GP or consultant. Patients are making the choice about which kinds of therapies they would like to consider for their particular problem and are then discussing these issues with a CAM practitioner.

They feel empowered by choosing CAM whereas their perception of conventional medicine is that they, as the patient, have less input and indeed less control over the treatments prescribed. Most complementary practitioners are prepared to listen to all their patient's symptoms. This process of listening, understanding and then involving the patient in the decision-making process is what seems to be attractive.

So it is not just whether homeopathy works better than painkillers for headaches. An important part is taking control of your headaches, understanding why they may occur and then receiving a treatment that is based on that understanding.

## Models of illness

The assumptions within CAM seek to develop our own intuitive understanding of the illness process. For example, we may think a cancer developed because of a particularly stressful divorce or that the shock of the sudden death of someone near and dear caused our migraines. Although this may not be a cause of a particular problem as far as conventional medicine is concerned, it is helpful when using some of the assumptions that relate to CAM.

In general, the models of illness and thinking processes within complementary medicine are often far closer to our own intuitive models and processes. This is why we may find them easier to accept, even though they may be scientifically unproven.

## Hands-on therapies

Many of the CAM therapies, particularly acupuncture, massage, healing and the manipulative therapies, mean that practitioners actually put their hands on their patients. This, in conventional medicine, has often been replaced by a careful history, investigations and the prescription pad.

It is interesting to observe that doctors who have taken up acupuncture frequently find enormous personal satisfaction in doing something manual that relieves their patients' pain. This creates practitioner satisfaction with the therapy as well as enhancing the doctor's belief in acupuncture. If the doctor then approaches patients with a technique about which he or she is very enthusiastic, this will inevitably be transmitted to those receiving the treatment and will, in all probability, improve the effects of that treatment.

## Do people get what they expect from CAM?

By and large, people seek out complementary practitioners through a series of informal networks. In practice, this often means asking friends and family, and sometimes their own GP, about a suitable practitioner. Recommendations are usually based on someone's previous experience of effective therapy.

The few surveys that have looked at consumer satisfaction with the treatment they have received have been positive. Most people receiving treatment appear to be very satisfied. This undoubtedly makes people in general view CAM more positively.

## KEY POINTS

- ✓ CAM focuses on an individualised approach to illness
- ✓ Most CAM therapies have their own unique approach to diagnosis and treatment
- ✓ CAM considers the whole person not individual symptoms

# Acupuncture

Acupuncture has probably been practised in China for around 3,500 years, but the exact date of its origin is difficult to determine. The first medical textbook on acupuncture was called the *Nei Ching Su Wen*; this literally means *The Yellow Emperor's Classic of Internal Medicine* and it dates from about 400 BC.

Acupuncture has been known to Western doctors since the Jesuits first went to China in the seventeenth century, and it was used extensively by physicians in this country in the early part of the nineteenth century. The first edition of *The Lancet* in 1823 carried a detailed report of the use of acupuncture in tympany (ear infections and/or deafness) and rheumatism, praising the virtues of this technique. The author, John Elliotson, was a consultant physician at St Thomas' Hospital in central London.

## Traditional Chinese medicine

The first recorded therapeutic success with acupuncture occurs in the 'historical records' of some 2,000 years ago. Pein Chueh, a physician, used acupuncture to revive a dying patient already in a coma. The practice of acupuncture was progressively developed and refined throughout Chinese history until the Ching dynasty (AD 1644–1911). During this period, acupuncture fell into disrepute and was discouraged in favour of Western medicine. However, since the Communist revolution of 1948 acupuncture has been revitalised and is now widely used in China.

Acupuncture is one of the therapeutic techniques used in traditional Chinese medicine (TCM), which has its own complete system of anatomy, physiology and diagnosis: the main concepts are described in detail in the *Nei Ching Su Wen*. The traditional Chinese viewed the human body as a balance between two opposing forces, yin and yang: yin represents placidity or water, whereas yang represents activity or fire. If yin or yang is deficient or in gross excess, the balance between them is distorted and disease results.

The Chinese concept of health can best be defined as a normal fluctuating balance between yin and yang. Their system of diagnosis and therapy is designed to determine the imbalance of yin and yang and to correct it, therefore restoring the person's health. To produce this change, the Chinese insert needles into acupuncture points. Most of the important acupuncture points are on 14 channels running over the body, each representing an internal organ. Qi, or vital energy, is said to flow through these channels. In disease, the flow of qi is altered and the insertion of an acupuncture needle into an appropriate point is said to correct the flow of vital energy, therefore restoring the body to good health.

The Chinese also developed a sophisticated idea of physiology (how living organisms function), and specific functions were defined for each of the 12 main organs. The *Nei Ching Su Wen* states that: 'the heart fills the pulse with blood . . . And the force of the pulse flows into the arteries, and the force of the arteries ascends into the lungs.' This describes the double circulation of blood (first passing through the lungs then through the body) some

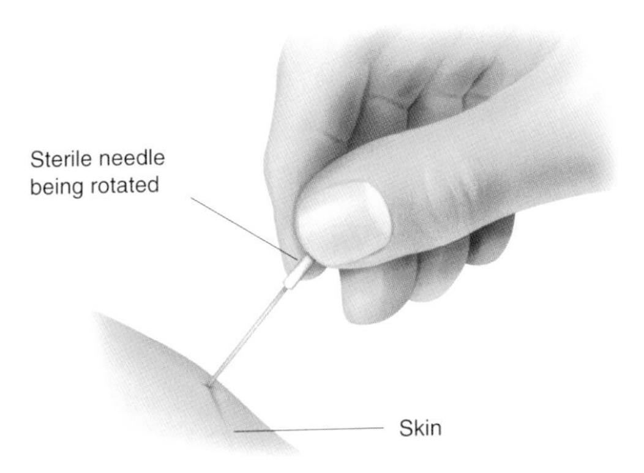


Acupuncture is a method of pain relief that involves insertion of fine sterile needles into specific points on the body. The needles are then rotated to produce stimulation.

2,000 years before the scientist William Harvey demonstrated the function of the heart and the circulation of blood in the seventeenth century.

The anatomy (acupuncture points and channels) and physiology of TCM, along with a detailed examination of the pulse and tongue, provide the basis for a TCM diagnosis. A practitioner then follows a set of empirical rules to select the appropriate acupuncture points to treat the disease and correct the imbalances (the pathogen).

Not all acupuncturists use a traditional Chinese approach. Some just treat the tender points that arise in various musculoskeletal diseases (such as arthritis). A number of clinical trials have shown that acupuncture in tender trigger points, which are also frequently acupuncture points, is effective for painful diseases.

In the treatment of pain, it is not yet clear which approach is best – the traditional Chinese diagnosis or simply treating tender trigger points. However, in non-painful diseases, such as asthma or irritable bowel syndrome, trigger points do not always occur, so to perform effective acupuncture a traditional diagnosis must be made and the points selected within the context of TCM.

## How does acupuncture work?

TCM practitioners can explain how and why acupuncture works and the underlying principles behind the selection of which points to treat, through their understanding of Chinese medicine. However, TCM is not firmly grounded in modern conventional science but there is considerable evidence to suggest that acupuncture points are important and special areas of the body, particularly in pain.

Research in the 1970s has shown clearly that over 70 per cent of trigger or 'ouch' points occurring in painful diseases were already defined as acupuncture points by the Chinese. Furthermore, many forms of therapy, particularly for diseases of the muscles, bones and joints, rely on the fact that stimulating or needling these trigger points can relieve pain.

We also know that acupuncture points have special electrical properties – they have a lower electrical resistance than the surrounding skin. However, no scientific evidence has yet been provided to prove (or disprove) the existence of the channels.

Acupuncture is used in the West primarily for painful conditions. Most research into the mechanism of acupuncture has been in this area. The gate control theory, developed by Melzack and Wall in

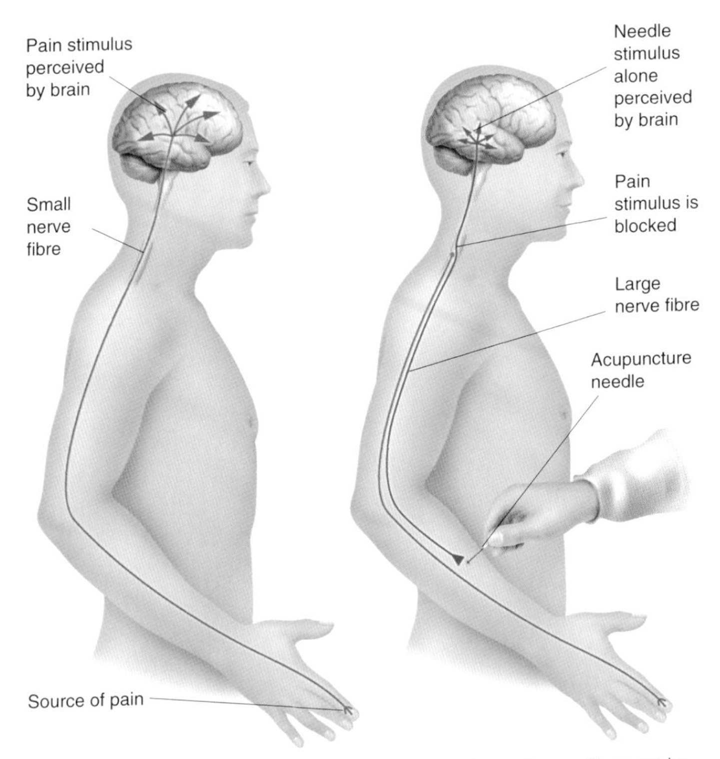


The gate control theory explains that the input of pain via small nerve fibres can be inhibited within the spinal cord by the stimulation of large nerve fibres with needles. Acupuncture can 'close the gate' to pain and block pain perception in the brain.

1965, explains that the input of pain via small nerve fibres can be inhibited within the spinal cord by the stimulation of large nerve fibres. Acupuncture has been shown to stimulate certain kinds of nerve fibres, thereby 'closing the gate' to pain and blocking pain perception.

The discovery of endorphins and enkephalins (the body's own natural opiate painkillers) has also strengthened the position of acupuncture as a treatment for pain. A number of studies have shown that acupuncture causes the release of these opiates into various areas of the nervous system.

Although there is good evidence for the mechanisms underlying the effect of acupuncture in both acute and chronic pain, there are, to date, no theories that explain how acupuncture may work in non-painful conditions such as asthma.

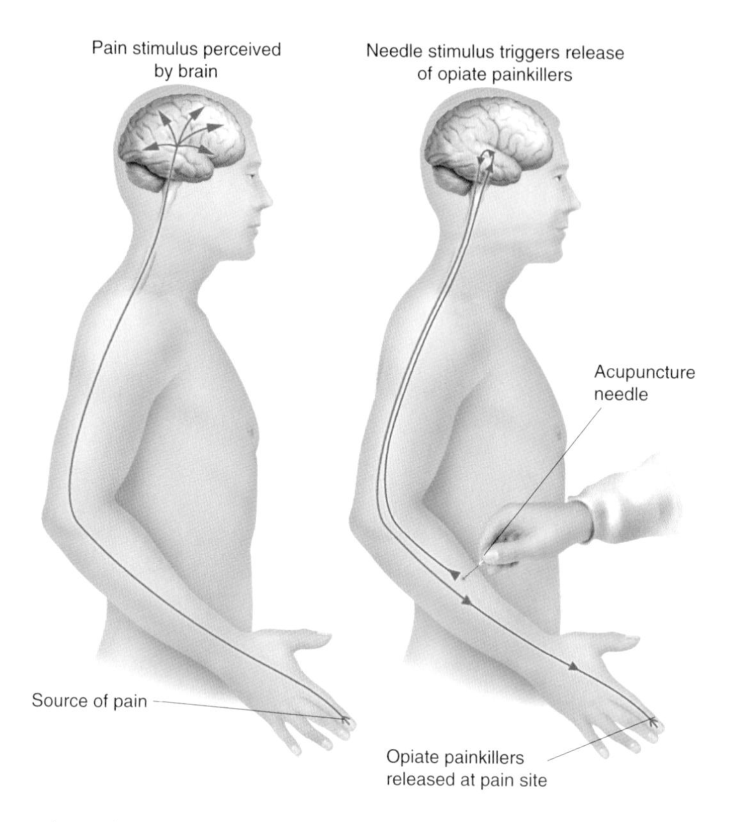


Acupuncture may cause the release of the body's own natural opiate painkillers into various areas of the nervous system.

## What does the treatment involve?

Needles are usually a few millimetres in diameter and, depending on the type of acupuncture used and the site of the problem, may be inserted at depths varying from a few millimetres to three to four centimetres. Six to ten needles will be used in each treatment session. The needles used should always be single-use, pre-sterilised, disposable needles which will be left in place for between 5 and 20 minutes. Sometimes a small electrical current is used to stimulate the needles. Before you receive any treatment, the acupuncturist will want to take a history to make a clear diagnosis of your condition. This may involve a traditional Chinese history as well as a Western diagnosis, depending on the approach used by, and techniques of, the acupuncturist.

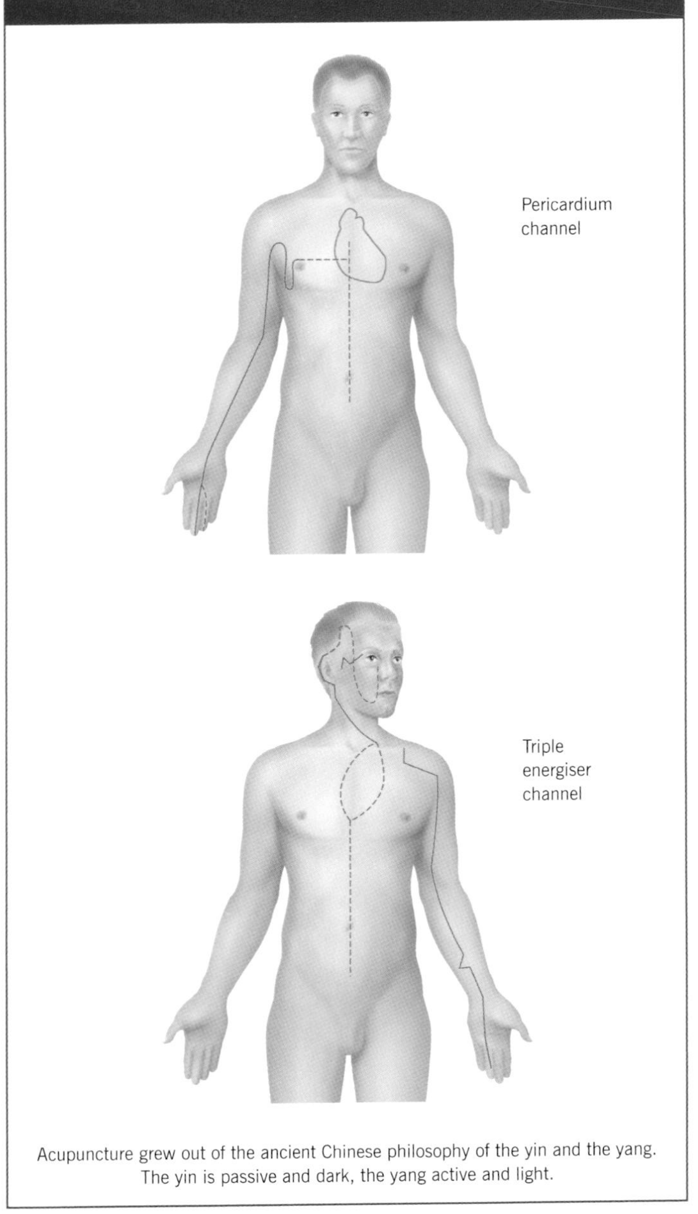

Acupuncture grew out of the ancient Chinese philosophy of the yin and the yang. The yin is passive and dark, the yang active and light.

## THE 12 PRIMARY ACUPUNCTURE MERIDIANS (contd)

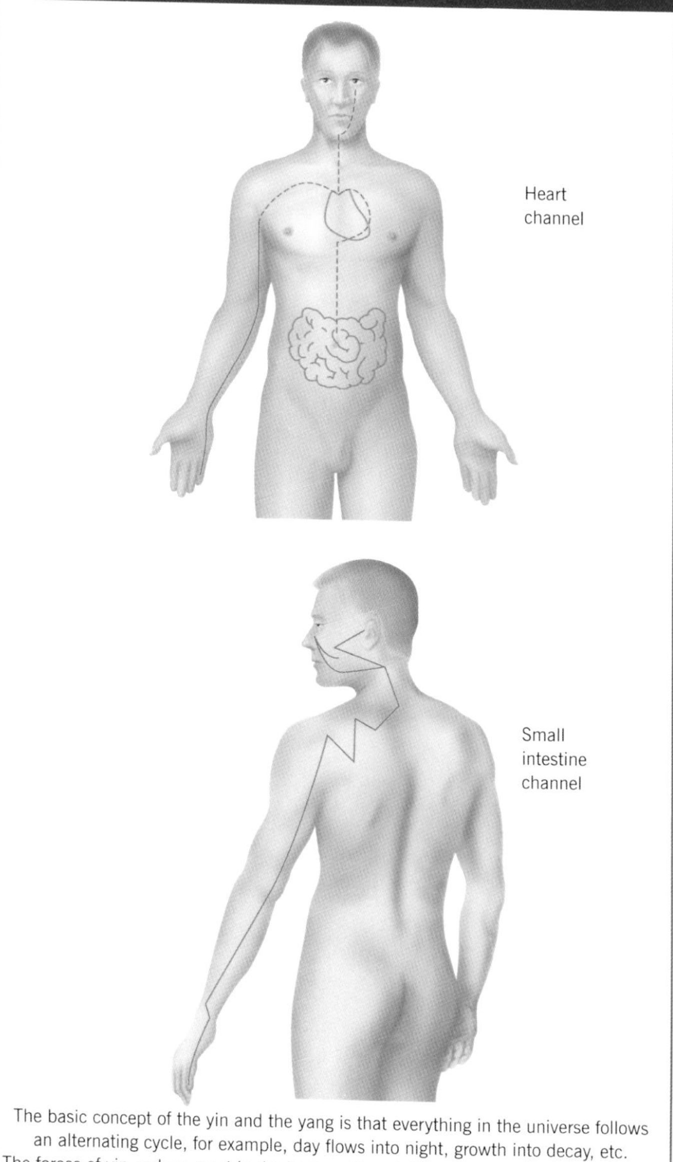


The basic concept of the yin and the yang is that everything in the universe follows an alternating cycle, for example, day flows into night, growth into decay, etc. The forces of yin and yang act in the body as they do throughout the natural universe.

## THE 12 PRIMARY ACUPUNCTURE MERIDIANS (contd)

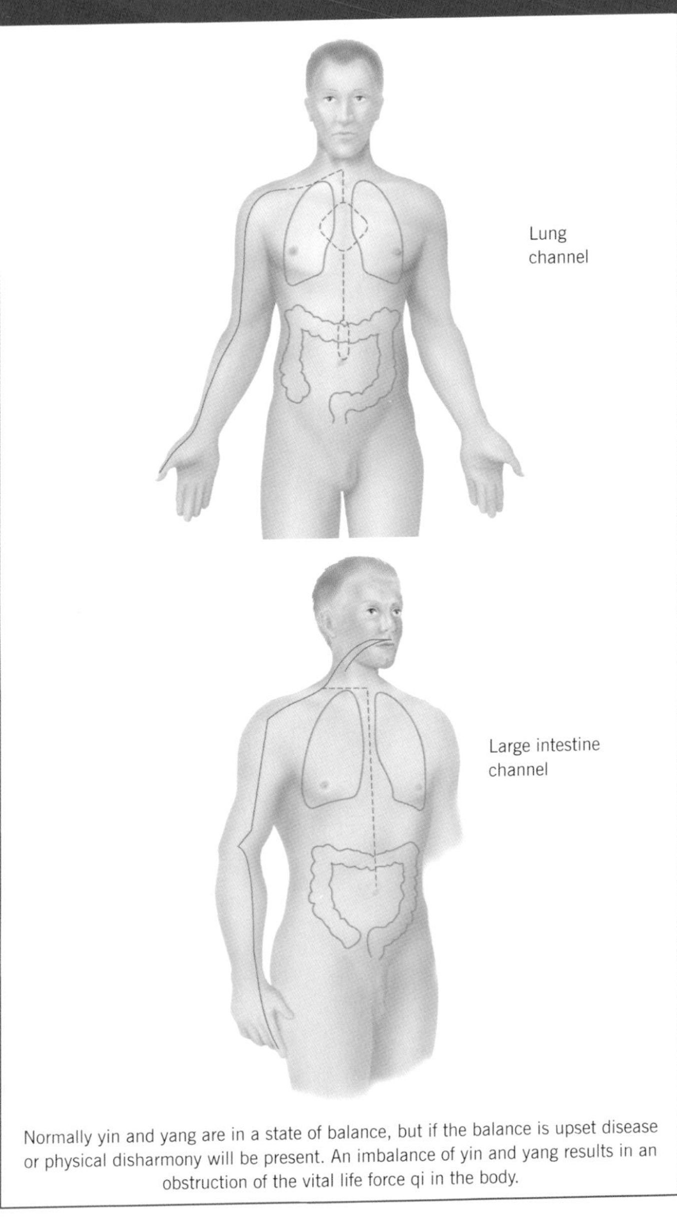


Normally yin and yang are in a state of balance, but if the balance is upset disease or physical disharmony will be present. An imbalance of yin and yang results in an obstruction of the vital life force qi in the body.

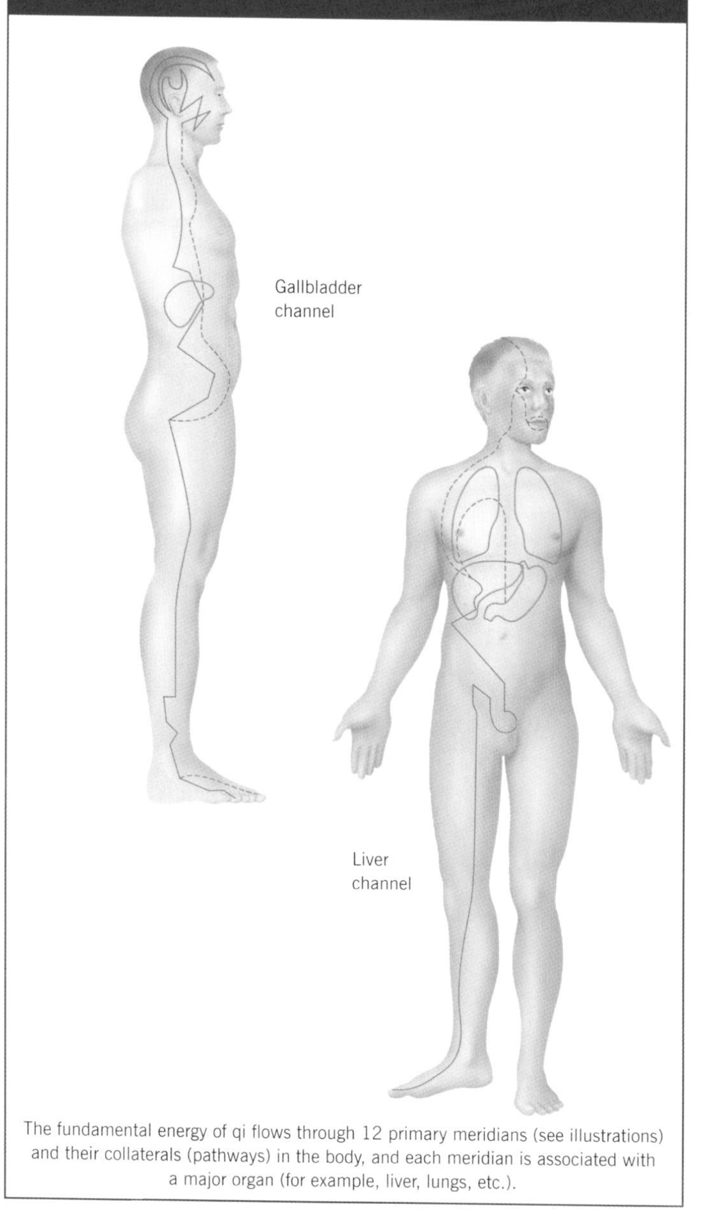

The fundamental energy of qi flows through 12 primary meridians (see illustrations) and their collaterals (pathways) in the body, and each meridian is associated with a major organ (for example, liver, lungs, etc.).

## THE 12 PRIMARY ACUPUNCTURE MERIDIANS (contd)

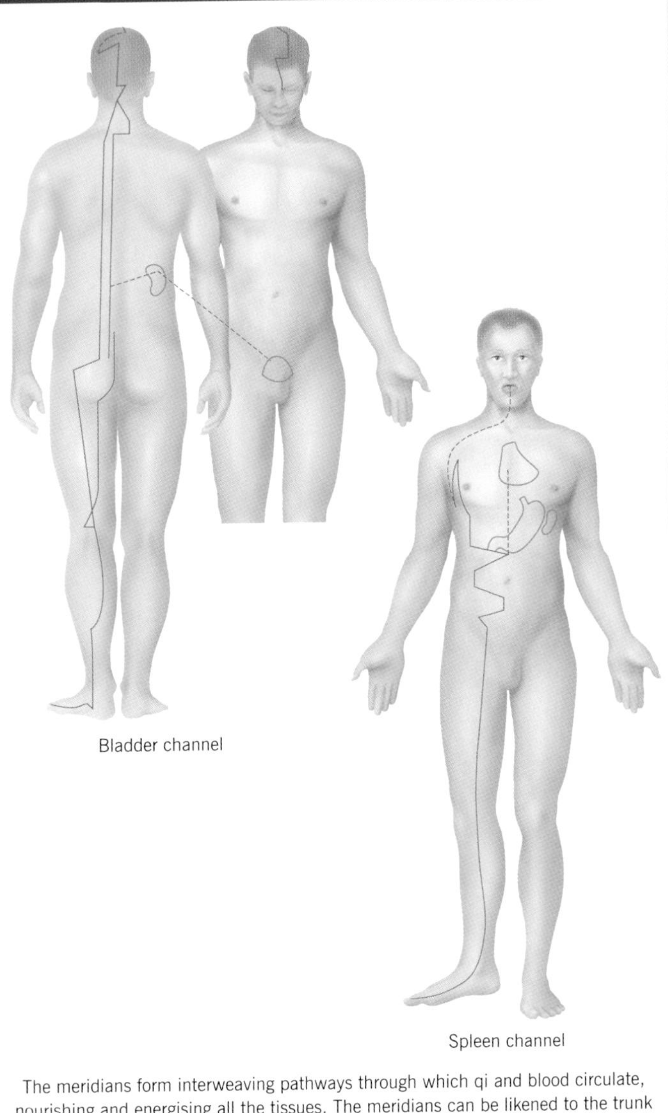

Bladder channel

Spleen channel

The meridians form interweaving pathways through which qi and blood circulate, nourishing and energising all the tissues. The meridians can be likened to the trunk of a tree whereas the collaterals are branches. The roots are represented by the organs and the sense organs by the leaves and flowers.

## THE 12 PRIMARY ACUPUNCTURE MERIDIANS (contd)

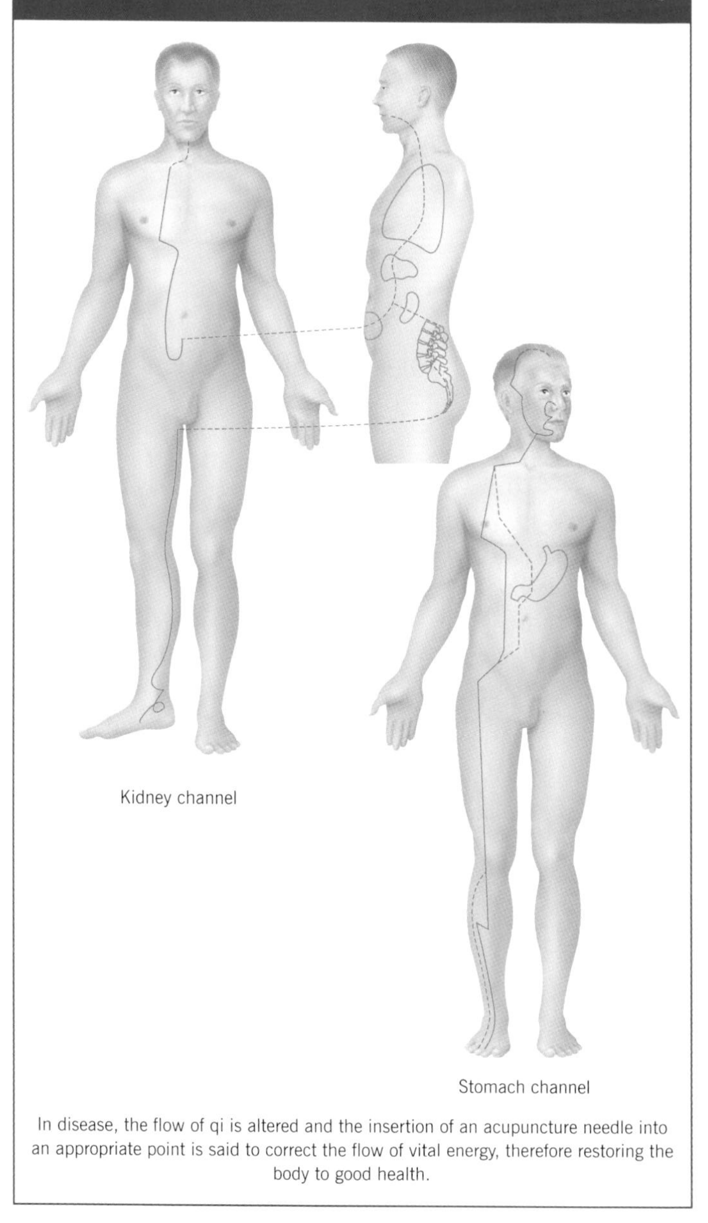

Kidney channel

Stomach channel

In disease, the flow of qi is altered and the insertion of an acupuncture needle into an appropriate point is said to correct the flow of vital energy, therefore restoring the body to good health.

In skilled hands, acupuncture treatment is relatively painless. After the treatment, you may notice a temporary worsening of your symptoms, but this usually indicates that you will experience an effective response later on. The treatment usually works in stages. The first one or two treatments may produce no effect or perhaps only a brief effect, and you will usually need a course of six to eight sessions for effective symptom relief. Once you have obtained relief, it often lasts for three to nine months. After this, one or two further treatments will 'top-up' the therapeutic benefit.

The acupuncturist will try to manipulate the needles so that you will feel a dull bursting or numb sensation around their site of insertion. This sensation is called 'de qi' (pronounced dar-chee) or 'obtaining energy' and traditionally it is suggested that 'de qi' may be an important part of the treatment process.

Sometimes your acupuncturist may use other methods of stimulating an acupuncture point, such as moxibustion – the burning of the dried herb wormwood (*Artemesia vulgaris*) just above the surface of the skin or on the end of a needle, or placing a cup over the acupuncture point.

## What can acupuncture treat?

Some acupuncture texts suggest that acupuncture is a universal system for treating almost all illnesses, but in the West it is primarily used for treating pain caused by problems in muscles, bones and joints. It may also be used to treat other illnesses such as migraine, irritable bowel syndrome or asthma. Acupuncture can also help to provide pain relief for people with cancer.

There has been quite a lot of research into acupuncture compared with some of the other complementary therapies. Research shows that it can help in headaches and migraine, dental pain and low back pain. Its use has also been well evaluated in the treatment of nausea (early morning sickness, post-anaesthetic nausea and the nausea caused by using powerful anti-cancer drugs).

There is some evidence that acupuncture may help to improve and accelerate recovery after a stroke. Although acupuncture does not appear to help people give up smoking, it can help overcome the withdrawal period from addiction to other, harder drugs.

Acupuncture may help people with asthma, although the evidence is a little uncertain at present. For many illnesses, the effect of acupuncture has still not been properly assessed.

## Is it safe?

Acupuncture is largely a safe treatment. A recent survey of 50,000 acupuncture treatments reported no serious adverse reactions. There are some fairly simple pieces of advice for anyone seeking acupuncture treatment.

First, you should go to a registered acupuncturist whose premises have been inspected and registered by the local health authority for the purpose of providing acupuncture. The health authority should be able to provide a list of these premises. This means that you will be given disposable (once-only use) acupuncture needles and there will be no danger of cross-infection, so you will not run the risk of picking up diseases.

If the acupuncturist is proposing to use an indwelling needle that may be left in place for a few days, then this may expose you to an increased risk of infection and is not a good idea, particularly if you have any problem with the valves of your heart.

There are also certain specific acupuncture points that should be avoided in pregnancy, although acupuncture in general is a very safe and effective treatment during pregnancy for both early morning sickness and pain.

## Whom should I see?

There are three main groups of acupuncturists: doctors, professional acupuncturists and physiotherapists.

The members of The British Medical Acupuncture Society are doctors and dentists. Their training usually involves several weekend acupuncture courses and is directed mainly at the treatment of pain. They may learn a small amount of TCM but most doctors in the UK will use Western acupuncture techniques.

Professional acupuncturists usually attend a three- or four-year training course, which may result in a university degree. These acupuncturists are well versed in the use of TCM and are registered with the British Acupuncture Council.

The Acupuncture Association of Chartered Physiotherapists also offers extensive training in TCM, a course that is fairly similar in detail to that attended by professional acupuncturists. However, many of its members use acupuncture more simply, to treat painful conditions as part of their physiotherapy practice.

These three organisations will provide you with detailed information about the acupuncturists available in your area (see Useful addresses, page 100).

## KEY POINTS

- ✓ Acupuncture is an ancient Chinese treatment system
- ✓ It is based on a traditional approach to diagnosis and treatment
- ✓ It is frequently used in chronic pain and works by changing our perception of pain in the nervous system
- ✓ Acupuncture is a safe treatment, usually requiring several sessions to achieve an effective result
- ✓ If you wish to receive this type of treatment, see a registered acupuncturist

# Healing

Healing or the 'laying on of hands' is one of the most ancient forms of health care and almost certainly the one in most widespread use in the UK. Some estimates suggest that there may be over 20,000 healers in the UK, although exact figures vary between 8,000 healers belonging to 16 different healing organisations and 14,000 healers registered as complementary practitioners.

Healing is probably best defined as the practice of conscious intentionality – that is, positive thinking and beliefs designed to

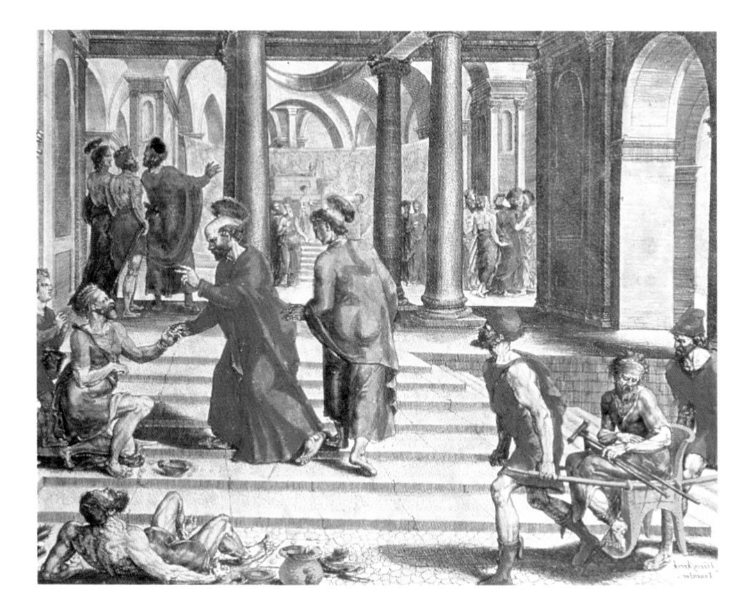

A sixteenth century engraving showing Saint Peter and Saint John healing a lame man.

improve the health and well-being of others. The origins of healing are probably very ancient, because they resemble certain Shamanistic practices which, if Australian Aboriginal culture is anything to judge by, have their origins in Neolithic societies. There are two features that all systems of healing share:

- There is usually some organised approach to the healing process. This may be religious (or recently 'New Age' spiritual beliefs) or may be linked to a particular system of medicine such as traditional Chinese medicine – for example, Qigong may be considered to be a system of healing firmly based on a traditional Chinese medical approach.
- Healers believe that they can somehow channel healing energy to the person being healed (the 'client').

Within Christian societies, healing became an important part of Christian ministry, particularly during mediaeval times when there were often few effective medicines. The UK has developed a strong healing tradition over the years and there are probably more healers working in the UK than in any other Western industrialised nation.

There are a variety of different approaches to healing:

- Lay healers describe themselves as being of no specific faith but have usually discovered some innate healing ability along with some concepts of helping to 'balance people's energy'.
- Spiritual healing is the specific laying on of hands and involves prayer and/or religious meditation.
- Reiki is a system of healing that involves an interactive approach where healing energy is transferred between the healer and the person being healed (the client) with the aim of restoring the client's energy balance.
- Therapeutic touch is a specific modern form of healing that was developed in the twentieth century by Professor Dolores Kreiger, an American nurse, to 'rebalance' or 'repattern' the 'energy field' of the client.

The mechanism involved in healing is unknown, but if healing works it must do so through an effect that encourages the client's own body to reverse the damage caused by their disease. In other words, the effect of the healer/client relationship actually promotes self-healing.

## What does healing involve?

The ways in which the various healing techniques may be practised vary enormously. There are some charismatic healers who have in the past been associated with celebrities and sportsmen. However, many healers work on an entirely voluntary basis with local people who contact them for help.

Healing may take place with the healer and client present in the same room at the same time, or it may be in the form of absent healing. In absent healing, the client may simply request that the healer prays or meditates for them at specific set times of the day.

Healing may be practised almost anywhere – including in doctors' surgeries, at special healing centres or in your home. A session may last from a few minutes to an hour and you may be treated in a sitting or lying position. Usually the healer will go through a quiet period, which is an initial preparation for them. During this time, they will relax and focus on your problem.

The healer may then pass his or her hands over your body, usually without touching you, and will try to identify the particular areas requiring healing. He or she may then either just leave the hands over the area of your body to heal it, or may move the hands in a stroking or sweeping manner over your body to rebalance your energy.

In general, healing is a soothing and relaxing experience and you may notice some degree of tingling or warmth around the area being healed. Some people experience quite remarkable help with just one or two healing sessions, whereas others need many sessions.

## Does healing work?

Healing may produce real benefit for people suffering from almost any illness. There have been a large number of clinical trials looking at different healing techniques. Probably the most thoroughly investigated technique is that of therapeutic touch, which by and large produces demonstrable benefit in a wide range of conditions. The evidence suggests that healing has a positive physiological effect on the body's healing process.

One of the most impressive studies, carried out in the early 1990s, involved the absent healing of about 1,000 patients admitted to an American intensive care unit after they had experienced chest pain. Patients were randomly allocated to two groups: those who received absent healing and those who did not, although the patients were unaware which group they were allocated to. The outcome of their stay in hospital was recorded independently by someone who did not know who had received treatment. The results were quite astonishing and suggested that the absent healing had caused a dramatic effect because people who had healing were more likely to survive and had fewer complications.

At present, it's difficult for conventional science to explain this phenomenon. The positive feelings that a person experiences in the presence of somebody who knows and cares about them very deeply may be part of the whole healing process. However, this doesn't explain absent healing.

## Is healing safe?

There have been no reported adverse physical reactions to healing. However, non-medical healers should not diagnose medical problems.

All responsible healing organisations suggest to their healers that they should work with conventional doctors and base their treatment firmly on a clear conventional diagnosis. This will avoid people with a disease that should be treated conventionally going to a healer who most likely will not have medical training and is not in a position to make diagnoses.

## Whom should I see?

There are two main healing organisations in the UK, both of which have clear ethical and professional guidelines. The most important of these guidelines is that a healer should always work with those who have medical responsibility for the client and should respect the client's confidentiality. A clear code of ethics and a list of appropriately qualified individuals are available from the National Federation of Spiritual Healers and the Confederation of Healing Organisations (see Useful addresses, pages 101–2).

## KEY POINTS

- ✓ Healing involves the 'laying on of hands' or absent healing (for example, prayer), with the intention of alleviating illness and suffering
- ✓ Healing is in common use in the UK
- ✓ There are many different types of healing

# Herbal medicine

Herbal medicine uses plants for medicinal purposes. The term 'herb' includes leaves, stems, flowers, fruits, seeds, roots, rhizomes and bark, although in many traditions other naturally occurring substances including animal and mineral products are also used.

There can be little doubt that the use of plants for healing purposes is the most ancient form of medicine known. Men and women, led by instinct, taste, tradition and experience, used plants that were not part of their normal diet for healing purposes. The physical evidence for herbalism goes back some 60,000 years to a Neanderthal burial site uncovered in 1960 in the Middle East.

In China, Huang Di, the legendary Yellow Emperor, is credited with writing *The Yellow Emperor's Classic of Internal Medicine* in about 400 BC which lists 12 herbal prescriptions. The authorship of China's first *Materia Medica (Shen Nong Ben Cao Jing)* is credited to the mythical Shen Nong ('divine father'), the Yellow Emperor's predecessor.

The Egyptians are also renowned for the use of herbs, and official schools for herbalists existed in Egypt as early as 3000 BC. The *Ebers Papyrus*, written around 1500 BC and discovered in 1862, contains around 876 prescriptions made up of more than 500 different substances.

Many of the founders of the ancient Greek schools of medicine apparently owed their learning to the Egyptians. Hippocrates was tutored by Egyptian priest-doctors, and his writings mention over 250 medicinal plants.

A vast body of Greco-Roman

knowledge of herbs was preserved and enlarged upon by the Arabs. This knowledge, much of which had been lost to Europe in the Dark Ages, was reintroduced to Europe when the Crusaders returned from the Middle East.

In India too, traditional medicine incorporated a large number of herbal remedies. The Indian *Materia Medica*, published in 1908, listed 2,982 medicinal plants.

During the eighteenth and nineteenth centuries, many Europeans emigrated to North America. These settlers discovered that the native American population was skilled at using the indigenous plants as medicines and they began to incorporate them into their own remedies. Many of these new herbal remedies from the Americas were also brought back to Europe.

Despite the popularity of herbalism in the West, by the beginning of the nineteenth century herbal medicine had begun to fall out of favour with the medical profession, which considered it to be unscientific and imprecise. In Britain, professional herbalism survived only through the establishment of the National Institute of Medical Herbalists in 1864, which is still flourishing today and is the oldest register of practising medical herbalists in the world.

## Herbal traditions

There are three main methods through which herbal medicines are prescribed: Chinese, Ayurvedic and Western.

Herbal medicines are an essential part of traditional Chinese medicine (TCM) and are prescribed according to an individualised diagnosis, much as one would prescribe particular acupuncture points. Ayurvedic herbs are prescribed according to the main underlying principles of Ayurvedic medicine, also on an individual basis. Western herbal prescriptions are individually formulated and usually involve a mixture of herbs.

Western herbal remedies are prepared solely from plant material, whereas traditional Chinese and Ayurvedic herbs may also use some animal and mineral substances. Chinese herbs are usually prepared as decoctions, which means that the herbal mixtures are boiled and the liquid is used medicinally. Ayurvedic and Western herbs are usually administered in tinctures (alcohol/water extracts). Many standard or patented traditional Chinese herbal products are available as pills, as are an increasing number of Western herbs.

Herbal preparations are available in health food shops and over the counter from pharmacies to treat a variety of quite specific medical problems (for instance, the use of St John's wort in depression).

## How does herbal medicine differ from conventional medicine?

Many conventional drugs come from the purified extracts of herbs, and both herbal and conventional medicines work through the same biochemical and physiological pathways. However, herbalists claim that one of the great strengths of using the unrefined whole plant is that the active ingredient is present with a number of other naturally occurring plant chemicals. This can make the action of the active ingredient far safer, reducing the chance of unpleasant side effects. For example, the herb meadowsweet contains both an aspirin-like substance and a stomach-soothing compound that could, in theory, prevent the indigestion that aspirin can cause. These views are attractive, but as yet unproven.

Herbalists tend to use many herbs together. The combinations are largely based on clinical experience rather than rigorous science. It seems that conventional medicine is trying to decrease the number of drugs given to people, whereas in herbal medicine sometimes the opposite occurs.

As with many other forms of complementary medicine, the prescription of a specific herb or mixture of herbs is based not only on a conventional medical diagnosis but also on the traditional diagnostic system that underpins the herbal prescription. For instance, a herb may be prescribed to strengthen the kidney or liver or to dispel heat.

## Does herbal medicine work?

Herbal medicines have been used widely for a large number of conditions over many thousands of years. Herbalists tend to treat chronic, benign conditions such as allergic disease (asthma and eczema), hormonal problems such as menopausal symptoms, premenstrual syndrome and painful, irregular or difficult periods, headaches (including migraine), irritable bowel syndrome and arthritis (both rheumatoid and osteoarthritis).

In practice, many herbalists combine their suggested herbal remedies with dietary recommendations and nutritional supplements. The aim of herbal medicine, particularly in these chronic, persistent complaints, is generally to improve well-being, and perhaps slow down or modify the natural history of an illness. Herbs can also be used to relieve depression or help sleep.

## What does the treatment involve?

Treatment by a herbalist will usually involve a detailed consultation to

## WHAT CAN HERBAL MEDICINE USEFULLY TREAT?

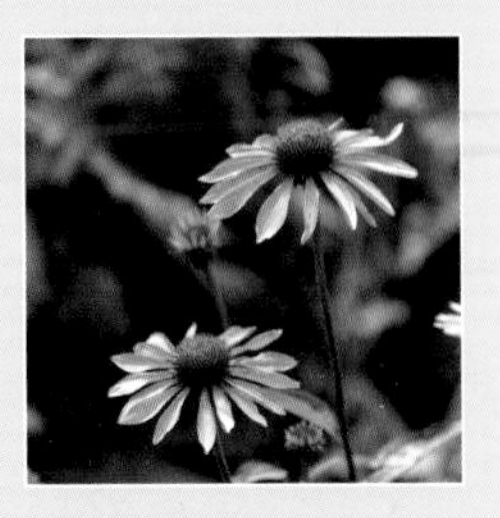

**Echinacea root (American coneflower root) (*Echinacea angustifolia, E. pallida, E. purpurea*)**

The use of echinacea in the treatment of bacterial and viral infections is well established and there has been much research interest in the stimulation of the immune system by this plant.

Taking echinacea persistently as a preventive measure seems to work far less well than taking it when you have an acute infection.

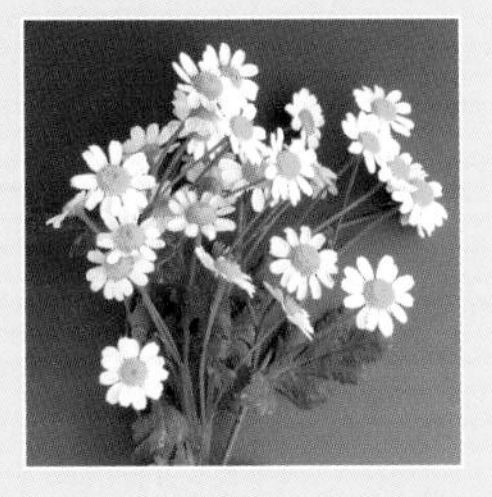

**Feverfew *(Tanacetum parthenium)***

Several clinical studies have demonstrated the effectiveness of feverfew in preventing migraine attacks.

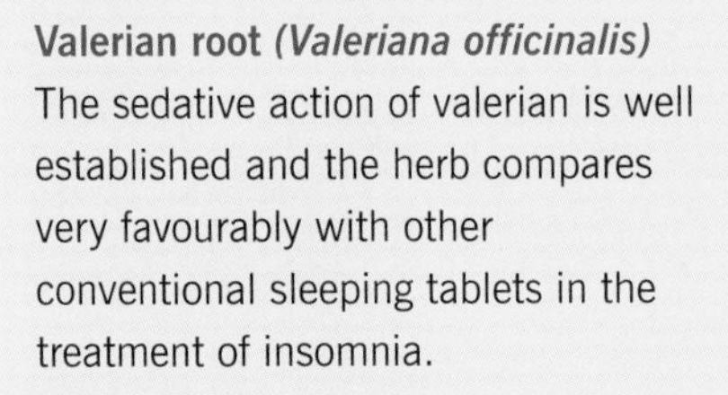

**Valerian root *(Valeriana officinalis)***

The sedative action of valerian is well established and the herb compares very favourably with other conventional sleeping tablets in the treatment of insomnia.

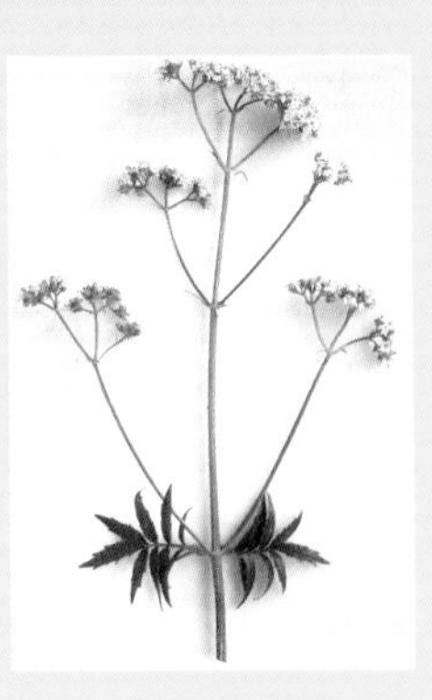

## WHAT CAN HERBAL MEDICINE USEFULLY TREAT? (contd)

**Ginkgo *(Ginkgo biloba)***

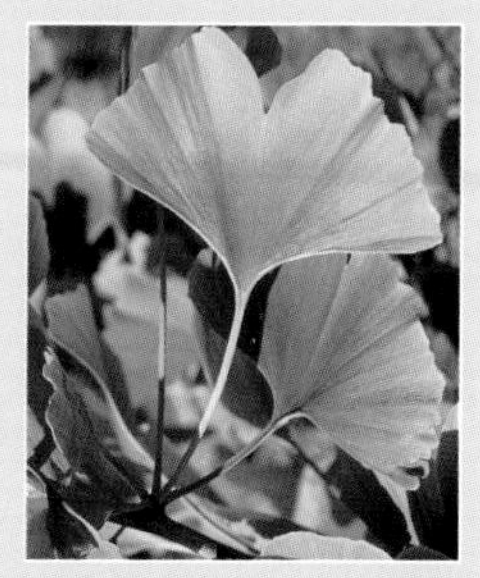

The main uses for *Ginkgo biloba* are for diseases of the circulatory system, particularly peripheral vascular disease in which the arteries are narrowed by deposits of fat in the arterial wall. *Ginkgo biloba* can also help to improve circulation in the brain and has been used to treat both depression and Alzheimer's disease with some degree of success. In Western countries, standardised extracts from the leaves are available in tablet, liquid and intravenous formulations, and in France and Germany these extracts are among the most commonly prescribed medications.

**Milk thistle *(Silybum marianum)***

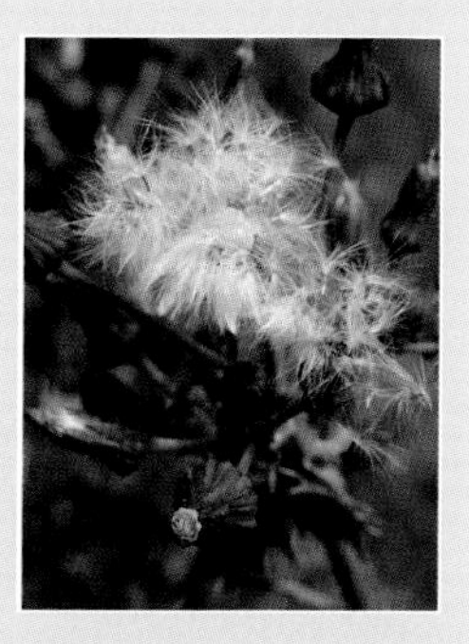

The seeds of milk thistle have been used medicinally for over 2,000 years. This herb is useful in a whole range of liver and gallbladder conditions.

## WHAT CAN HERBAL MEDICINE USEFULLY TREAT? (contd)

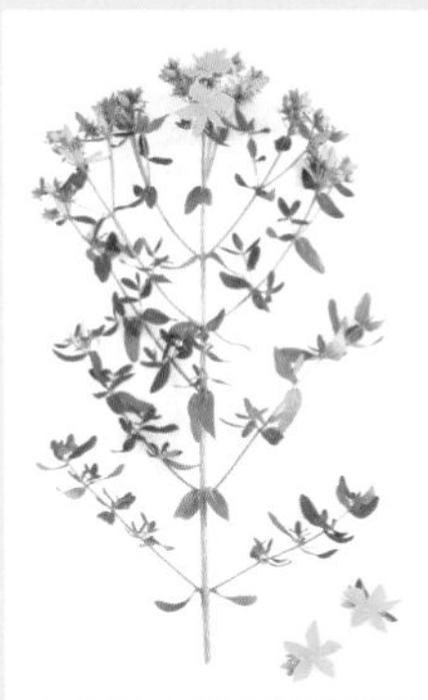

### St John's wort *(Hypericum perforatum)*

St John's wort has long been used for its anti-inflammatory, mild sedative and painkilling properties, although recent research has demonstrated that it does have some antiviral properties too. St John's wort has caught the public interest as the 'natural answer to Prozac', and there is no doubt from the clinical trials available that it acts very effectively as a mild antidepressant.

### Ginger *(Zingiber officinale)*

Ginger has been shown to have a number of actions, but it is probably best known for its effects in reducing nausea and vomiting. There has been considerable interest in this because it has few side effects compared with conventional anti-emetics (anti-nausea medicines).

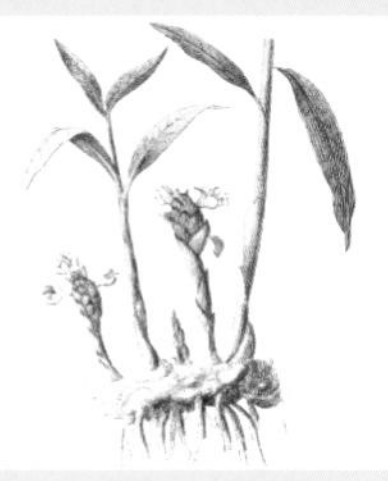

Ginger plant

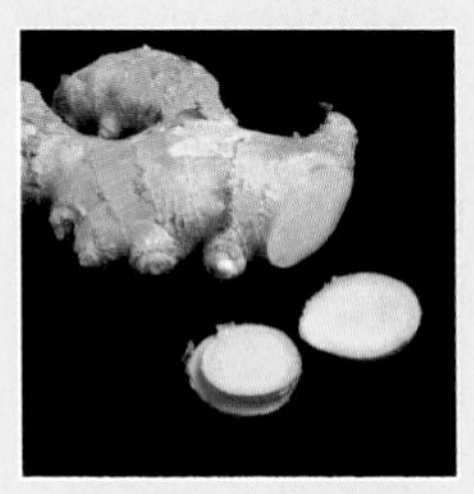

Ginger root

### Chinese herbal remedies

Chinese herbal mixtures have been shown to be particularly useful in the treatment of eczema, especially childhood eczema.

find out all your symptoms and your constitutional make-up. Herbs will then be prescribed based on the diagnosis made by the herbalist.

Treatment usually involves drinking a number of herbal extracts in teas or small amounts of alcohol that need to be taken at regular intervals, usually two to four times a day, over four to six weeks. The herbalist will usually review your clinical progress on a monthly basis. In general, you should begin to see some improvement in a long-term chronic problem within four to six months of taking herbal remedies.

## Is it safe?

The safety of herbal remedies has been the subject of much controversy. Herbal medicines must be produced using good manufacturing practice and must be free from adulteration. Medicines manufactured in the Westernised industrial nations or grown by herbalists themselves are almost certainly unadulterated.

Problems may occur with some patented medicines imported from Asia and the Far East, or sometimes with the pure herbal products, which may not be always as pure as one might expect and drugs (for example, steroids) have sometimes been detected. There are case reports of fatal events occurring when herbal products have been taken inappropriately. There was an outbreak of kidney disease after 'Chinese herbs' were prescribed by a slimming clinic in Belgium around 10 years ago, because the herbs had been unknowingly adulterated with a poisonous plant.

Herbs may also interact with conventional medicines. Some of the known interactions between herbal preparations and conventional drugs are described in the table. Always tell your herbal practitioner about all the conventional medicines that you are taking.

The National Institute of Medical Herbalists and the Register of Chinese Herbal Medicine take a very serious, and indeed very professional, view about the potential for adverse reactions with herbs. They have developed a system for reporting adverse reactions to herbs and these are being collated and recorded at the University of Exeter. The National Poisons Unit has also set up a database to record adverse herbal events.

You should be aware that taking a herbal remedy may cause an adverse reaction. If you think you are suffering from unexpected symptoms that may be produced by the herbal remedy you are taking, speak either with your own doctor or pharmacist (if the herbal remedy was self-prescribed) or with the herbal practitioner who prescribed the remedy.

## IMPORTANT POTENTIAL INTERACTIONS BETWEEN HERBAL AND CONVENTIONAL MEDICINES

| Herb | Conventional medicine | Potential problem |
|---|---|---|
| Echinacea (used for more than eight weeks) | Anabolic steroids, methotrexate, amiodarone, ketoconazole | Liver damage |
| Feverfew | Non-steroidal anti-inflammatory drugs (such as ibuprofen) | Inhibition of herbal effect |
| Feverfew, garlic, ginseng, ginkgo, ginger | Warfarin | Altered blood clotting times |
| Ginseng | Phenelzine sulphate | Headache, tremulousness, manic episodes |
| Ginseng | Oestrogens, corticosteroids | Additive effects |
| St John's wort | Monoamine oxidase inhibitor (MOI) and serotonin reuptake inhibitor (SRI) antidepressants may interact with the oral contraceptives and anticoagulants (do not take together) | Mechanism of herbal effect uncertain Insufficient evidence of safety with other antidepressants; ineffective contraception and anticoagulation |
| Valerian | Barbiturates | Additive effects, excessive sedation |
| Kyushin, liquorice, plantain, uzara root, hawthorn, ginseng | Digoxin | Interference with normal action |

## IMPORTANT POTENTIAL INTERACTIONS BETWEEN HERBAL AND CONVENTIONAL MEDICINES (contd)

| Herb | Conventional medicine | Potential problem |
|---|---|---|
| Evening primrose oil, borage | Anti-epilepsy drugs | Lowered seizure threshold |
| Shankapulshpi (Ayurvedic preparation) | Phenytoin | Inhibition of drug effect |
| Echinacea, zinc (immuno-stimulants) | Immunosuppressants (such as corticosteroids, cyclosporin) | Antagonistic effects |
| St John's wort, saw palmetto | Iron | Tannic acid content of herbs may limit iron absorption |
| Kelp | Thyroxine | Iodine content of herb may interfere with thyroid replacement |
| Liquorice diuretic | Spironolactone | Antagonism of effect |
| Karela, ginseng | Insulin, sulphonylureas, biguanides | Altered glucose concentrations – these herbs should not be prescribed in patients with diabetes |

Data from: Miller LG. Herbal Medicinals: Selected clinical considerations focusing on known or potential drug–herb interactions. *Archives of Internal Medicine* 1998; vol. 158: pp. 2200–2211.

## WHOM SHOULD I SEE?

Herbalists work largely in their own small private practices, or in association with other complementary practitioners in clinics. Few herbalists work within the NHS.

There are two main organisations for herbalists: the National Institute of Medical Herbalists and the Register of Chinese Herbal Medicine. These bodies act as the regulatory and registering bodies in herbal medicine. Most herbalists in this country have taken a three- or four-year training course in herbal medicine and this has enabled them to pass an examination to become a member of the National Institute of Medical Herbalists. If they have skills in traditional Chinese herbalism, these have usually been added after their initial Western herbal training.

Some acupuncturists use traditional Chinese herbs as part of their practice. Their training is firmly grounded in traditional Chinese medicine, and combines herbal medicine and acupuncture in the same way as in the practice of Chinese-trained traditional Chinese doctors. There are a small number of medically qualified practitioners who are trained to prescribe herbal remedies.

If you are thinking of seeing a herbalist, he or she should be a member of the National Institute of Medical Herbalists or the Register of Chinese Herbal Medicine (see Useful addresses, page 102).

## KEY POINTS

- ✓ Herbal medicine involves the use of plant extracts to treat illness
- ✓ See a registered herbalist
- ✓ Be careful of interactions between conventional medicines and herbs, and tell your herbalist and your GP exactly what you are taking

# Homeopathy

The word homeopathy is derived from two Greek words: *homoios*, meaning similar, and *pathos*, meaning suffering. The combination of these two words defines the practice of homeopathy. The main governing principle of this form of medicine is summed up by the Latin phrase *simila, similibus curentur* – like cures like.

This approach contrasts with the principles of conventional medicine, which are allopathic – the Greek word *allos* meaning different. An appropriate remedy produces symptoms different (or opposite) from those of the disease – for instance, the suppression of a fever by aspirin.

'Like cures like' means, simply, that a homeopathic substance producing certain symptoms in a healthy person will treat similar symptoms in an ill person. For example, the medicine *Belladonna* (deadly nightshade, atropine) causes mania and confusion, a flushed red face, dilated pupils, a high fever and a dry mouth. If a person had similar symptoms, for instance as a result of an infection, a homeopath would assume that a tiny dose of *Belladonna* could relieve the complaint. In other words, a homeopath can use the toxic effects as a symptom 'picture', to select the appropriate medication.

## Principles of homeopathy

The basic principles of homeopathy were first defined by the German physician Dr Samuel Hahnemann (1755–1843). He seems to have based many of his original thoughts on Hippocratic principles that suggested symptoms were an expression of nature's healing powers. Another German physician,

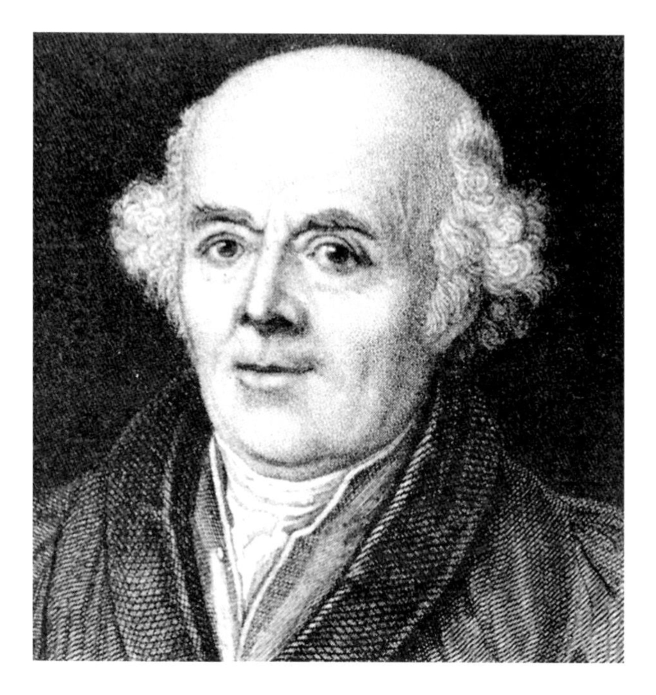

Dr Samuel Hahnemann (1755–1843), German physician and pioneer of homeopathy.

George Stahl, also stumbled across and used homeopathic principles about a century before Hahnemann's birth.

Hahnemann developed homeopathy by carefully observing in detail the effects of specific medicines, both in healthy people and in ill people. The first clearly defined by him was that of Peruvian cinchona bark (quinine). During the eighteenth century, this remedy was commonly used to treat many infections, including malaria and intermittent fever. On dosing himself up with cinchona bark, Hahnemann found that he was able to mimic many of the symptoms of malaria. It occurred to him that the bark reduced this febrile (fever-producing) disease by producing its own self-limiting fever. Similarly, mercury was used as a treatment for syphilis, and Hahnemann noted that mercurial fever was in many ways similar to the symptoms of early syphilis.

Hahnemann began to test other substances. He either took them himself or one of his friends or students took them. He made detailed records (drug pictures) of the mental and physical symptoms that occurred over the following week or two. It is important to understand that homeopathic prescribing is as much based on mental symptoms as it is on physical complaints.

Hahnemann slowly began to build a detailed 'library' of drug pictures, each drug being associated with a long list of symptoms. If you require any homeopathic treatment, a detailed history will be taken, so that your symptoms can be fitted into the most appropriate drug picture and the required remedy can be prescribed.

More recently, the prescription of homeopathic drugs has tended to be divided into two main approaches: the constitutional and the symptomatic. Constitutional remedies are designed to rebalance you as a whole – your body, mind and emotions. For instance, if you suffer from recurrent attacks of indigestion, you may be given a remedy based on your general manner and personality, with the idea of controlling both your symptoms and their cause in the long term. Symptomatic prescribing is based on your immediate presenting symptoms and is usually effective in controlling acute and minor illnesses such as colds. Constitutional and symptomatic remedies are sometimes given together to obtain the best therapeutic results.

Homeopathic pharmacies (particularly in Europe) have also developed 'complex' homeopathic preparations. These are effectively mixtures of several homeopathic remedies, all of which may be indicated in different people for the same group of symptoms.

## Homeopathic preparations

Homeopathic medicines are made from naturally occurring substances and are so dilute that they frequently contain none of the original substance.

The manufacture of homeopathic medicines involves two techniques: dilution and succussion. The homeopath dilutes the medicines in two main ways – decimal or D (one drop of tincture in 10 drops of water) and centesimal or C (one drop of tincture in 100 drops of water). For example, 30C is the original mother tincture diluted one in a hundred, 30 times. Between each dilution, it is necessary actively to shake the medication for a period of at least 10 seconds. This agitation, or succussion, appears to be an essential part of what makes homeopathic medicines effective. Usually only a small drop of

## HOW HOMEOPATHIC REMEDIES ARE MADE

The original material must be broken down so its essence can be extracted and dissolved in alcohol/water

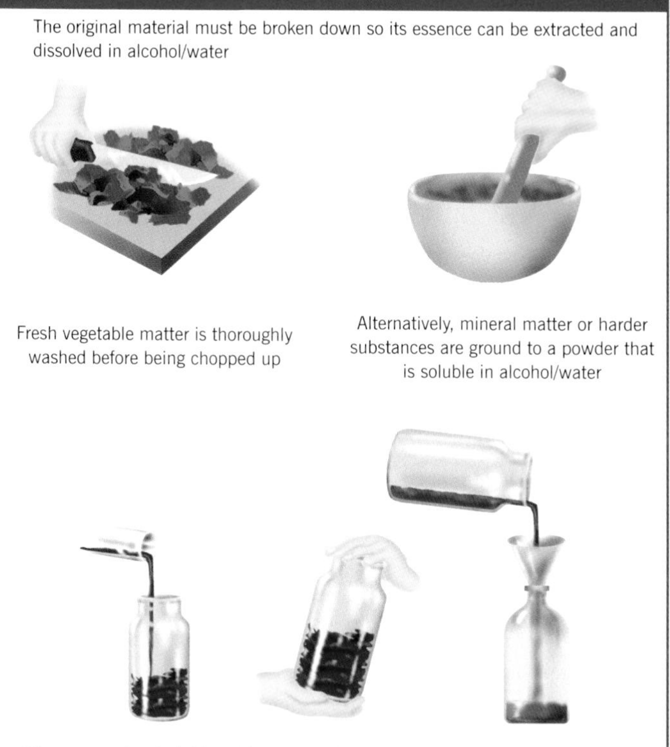

Fresh vegetable matter is thoroughly washed before being chopped up

Alternatively, mineral matter or harder substances are ground to a powder that is soluble in alcohol/water

The prepared material is put into a sealable jar and an alcohol/water mixture is added. The jar is then sealed with an airtight lid and the contents shaken vigorously (successed). The mixture may be allowed to stand for up to four weeks, being shaken occasionally. The 'mother tincture' is strained into a clean vessel.

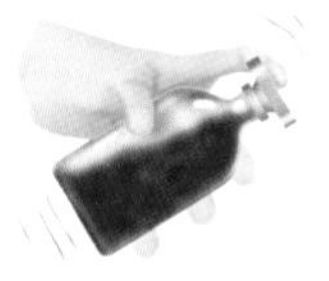

The mother tincture is diluted either 1:10 or 1:100 (mother tincture: alcohol/water mixture) and successed (shaken vigorously)

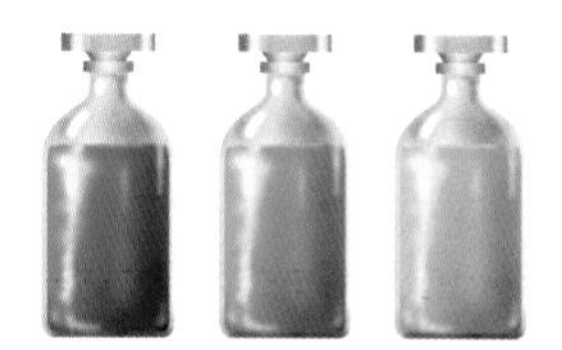

The mixture is diluted and successed repeatedly. Between each dilution it is necessary to shake the mixture for at least 10 seconds

medicine is taken once or twice a day, the exact dose dependent on the dilution being used.

In conventional medicine, when you are prescribed a drug, you are usually given large doses. This tends to work on the principle that the bigger the dose the greater the therapeutic effect. Homeopathic prescribing, however, adopts the opposite view: the smaller the drug dose, the more potent its effect.

## Does homeopathy work?

There has been quite a lot of research into homeopathy and this can be divided roughly into three areas: animal studies, laboratory experiments and clinical trials.

An example of an animal study is looking at whether homeopathic medicines added to the drinking water of farm animals may stop recurrent miscarriage in pigs or mastitis in cows. There have been relatively few animal studies but most have been positive and suggest that homeopathy is of therapeutic value.

A number of laboratory studies have also been performed looking at whether homeopathy can increase the excretion of toxic substances (for instance, arsenic) from poisoned plants and animals. Some studies have looked at the effect of homeopathy on specific reactions produced by enzymes in test tubes. Others have looked at the potential for homeopathy to inhibit or excite the growth of plants in certain specific conditions. These studies largely suggest that homeopathic preparations, even though they may be too dilute to contain any actual molecules of the original substances, have clear effects on biological systems.

Clinical trials have been conducted among patients being treated for certain conditions. People are allocated treatment at random and neither the patient nor the doctor knows who receives homeopathy and who receives a pill (placebo) that looks and tastes exactly the same. It does appear from these studies that homeopathy has an effect that is greater than a placebo (dummy treatment), although there's not enough clinical research to state categorically that homeopathy works in any specific condition.

Homeopathy cannot be recommended for any specific conditions. However, it is, in general, used to manage long-term chronic conditions as well as some acute self-limiting conditions like colds and flu. Recent studies suggest that, although homeopathy may be fairly comparable in effectiveness to conventional treatments for acute respiratory problems, the rate of side effects that occur in homeopathically treated patients is far lower.

## How does homeopathy work?

Most conventionally trained doctors find it difficult to imagine how homeopathy works. Indeed if homeopathy does work, then the mechanism involved challenges science's whole understanding of the body's biochemistry and physiology. So, as a consequence, homeopathy has, over the last 200 years, been the subject of intense and often hostile debate within medicine.

There have been suggestions that the process of serial dilution and succussion creates a 'memory of the substance' in the diluted water and alcohol mixtures. It is this 'memory within the water' that seems to contain the active therapeutic principle, but such suggestions are speculation rather than hard scientific evidence.

## What does treatment involve?

At your first session, a homeopath will take a very detailed history from you to establish a complete picture of your symptoms. Not only will they want to know your state of mind and the exact nature of your symptoms, they will also want to know what makes your symptoms better or worse. Having obtained a complete picture, the homeopath will then try to match your symptoms to a particular remedy. A prescription for a simple acute problem can sometimes be done over the telephone or in a very short period of time.

In chronic (long-lasting) conditions, it will usually be at least a month before the homeopath will review your situation. This is because homeopathic remedies take time to act. Sometimes, there will be an initial aggravation or healing crisis – this is frequently a good sign and indicates that the homeopathy might be effective. Usually the homeopathic remedy or remedies will need to be changed on several occasions during your course of treatment. You should allow at least a six-month period to elapse before you decide whether homeopathy is effective for you – particularly if you are seeking advice for a chronic condition.

While it is impossible to be specific about the type of conditions that can be helped by homeopathy, most homeopaths treat a wide range of problems. This includes allergic conditions (such as eczema and asthma), irritable bowel syndrome, migraine, gynaecological problems (such as painful periods and premenstrual syndrome), psychological problems (such as depression and anxiety) and arthritis.

The most important initial step before considering homeopathy is to make sure that you have, as far as possible, obtained a clear diagnosis from your doctor. You should also understand what conventional treatments are available to you so that you can consider whether homeopathy is an appropriate and reasonable approach to your condition.

## Is it safe?

Homeopathy can cause a flare-up of your original condition and this is usually considered by homeopaths to be part of the healing process. There is no evidence that homeopathy itself can cause serious or permanent adverse effects.

However, some homeopaths may suggest that you stop your conventional medicine as they say that this can interfere with the homeopathic treatment. This can be extremely dangerous in some conditions – so you should make sure you consult your own doctor before stopping any conventional medicines on the advice of a homeopath.

The essence of good integrated care is communication between those treating you, so that treatment does not put you at any risk.

## Whom should I see?

There are about 1,000 doctors practising homeopathy in the UK. Most of them are GPs and many will offer homeopathy as part of their general practice. The Faculty of Homeopathy of the General Medical Council is responsible for training and keeping a register of medically qualified homeopaths. Doctors may be Associates, Members or Fellows.

There are about 1,500 non-medically qualified homeopaths who work largely within the private sector. Training for homeopaths without a medical degree varies greatly but some do four years part-time and a few three years full-time. Some training courses leading to university degrees in homeopathy have recently been introduced. Non-medically qualified homeopaths can be contacted through the Society of Homeopaths (see Useful addresses, page 103).

## KEY POINTS

- ✓ Homeopathy was developed by Samuel Hahnemann 200 years ago in Germany
- ✓ It involves the use of dilute or infinitesimal amounts of various substances in solution for treating illness
- ✓ The symptoms produced by the homeopathically diluted substance in a healthy person can be matched with the symptoms of an ill person; this 'best match' remedy is then used to treat the illness – like cures like

# Manipulative medicine

Manipulation uses techniques designed to affect the musculoskeletal system (muscles, bones, joints and connective tissue) and is usually targeted mainly at the spine. The word manipulation is derived from the Latin word *manipulare*, 'to handle'. The use of manipulation can be dated to the writings of Hippocrates in Roman times. Galen (AD 131–202) describes how a lack of sensation and tingling in the fingers were cured by treatment of the neck.

Bone setters employing simple manipulative techniques were popular in both Europe and America in the nineteenth century. From these observations and experiences, the techniques of osteopathy and chiropractic developed in the USA. Both are fairly recent disciplines.

Osteopathy was developed by the American doctor Andrew Taylor Still (1828–1912), who believed that the spinal structure governed the health of the whole body. He developed a theory that misalignments of the bones in the spine were either the cause or the result of specific illnesses, and correcting the spinal abnormalities could cure almost all illnesses, including infections.

Daniel David Palmer developed chiropractic in 1895 in the USA. At the time he was a non-medically qualified 'magnetic' or hypnotic healer. He believed that the body was filled with a vital force, which he described as 'innate intelligence' and that correcting the misalignments or subluxations (partial dislocations) in the spine would enable the nervous system to work most efficiently and could cure almost any illness.

Both osteopathy and chiropractic had philosophical origins and practitioners believed that the 'life force' underpinned well-being. Although most modern manipulators no longer support these concepts but see their discipline more as a question of solving mechanical problems, some chiropractors and osteopaths still hold to the notion of a vital healing force.

## Who manipulates?

There are four professional groups who often use many of the manipulative techniques interchangeably: osteopaths, chiropractors, physiotherapists and medical practitioners.

Osteopaths and chiropractors are both statutorily registered and undergo four- or five-year full-time educational courses. Manipulation is also used widely by physiotherapists and medical practitioners. Physiotherapists usually learn simple manipulative techniques as part of their undergraduate course and can go on to develop this skill through various courses in their postgraduate training. Doctors, through organisations such as the British Institute of Musculoskeletal Medicine, can also learn manipulation and can obtain postgraduate qualifications as orthopaedic physicians.

It used to be the case that chiropractors tended to use more force with short, sharp, high-velocity manipulative thrusts, whereas osteopaths and physiotherapists would use gentler, more repetitive techniques best described as 'mobilisation'. Now the differences between the professions using manipulation have become blurred. Although osteopaths in the UK are solely manipulative, in the USA an osteopathic qualification is of equivalent status to a medical qualification and an osteopathic doctor might not use manipulation, but would in effect practise conventional medicine.

## Does manipulation work?

Various problems are said to respond to manipulation, although inevitably the scientific evidence lags behind the clinical recommendations made by most manipulators.

Spinal manipulation may help patients who have headaches and facial pains that may originate from their neck. Spinal pain, whether it is neck or low back pain, or pain referred from the spine into the tummy, pelvis or down the leg (sciatica) can also benefit. Sprains, strains, bursitis and 'tendonitis' in the hips, shoulders and peripheral joints may also respond.

GPs are recommended by their own Royal College to refer patients with uncomplicated low back pain (back pain that does not need a

**The spine – side view**

Viewed from the side the human spine has a definite curve. The spine is not a rigid structure; it is able to bend and flex because there are cushions or discs between each of the vertebrae. The vertebrae attach to the skull at the top and the pelvis at the bottom.

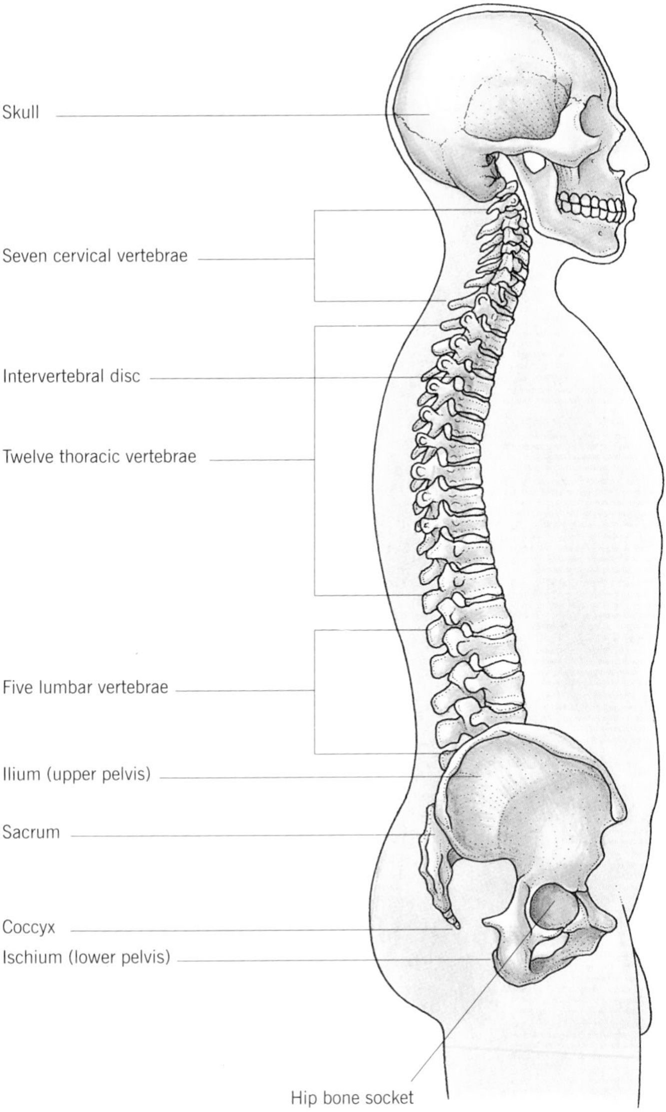

Skull

Seven cervical vertebrae

Intervertebral disc

Twelve thoracic vertebrae

Five lumbar vertebrae

Ilium (upper pelvis)

Sacrum

Coccyx

Ischium (lower pelvis)

Hip bone socket

**The spine – back view**

Viewed from the rear the human spine consists of a vertical column of bony blocks called vertebrae, which sit one on top of another. The vertebrae are numbered in descending order according to their location:

- Seven cervical vertebrae = C1–C7
- Twelve thoracic vertebrae = T1–T12
- Five lumbar vertebrae = L1–L5

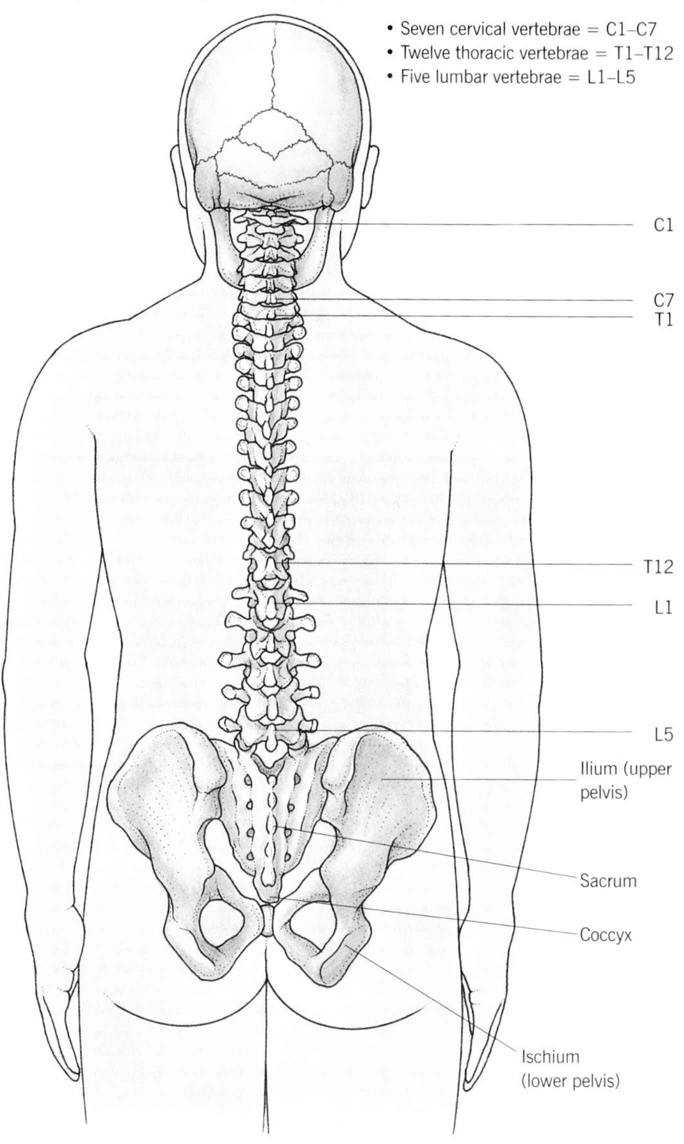

## MANIPULATIVE TECHNIQUES

The various manipulative techniques include the following:

- Soft tissue techniques, which involve stretching, movement or massage of muscles and ligaments.

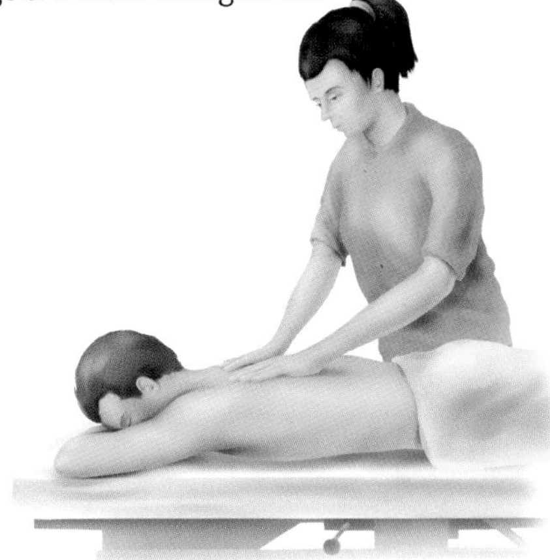

- Mobilisation, which involves the passive and gentle repetitive movement of a joint through its normal range of movement.

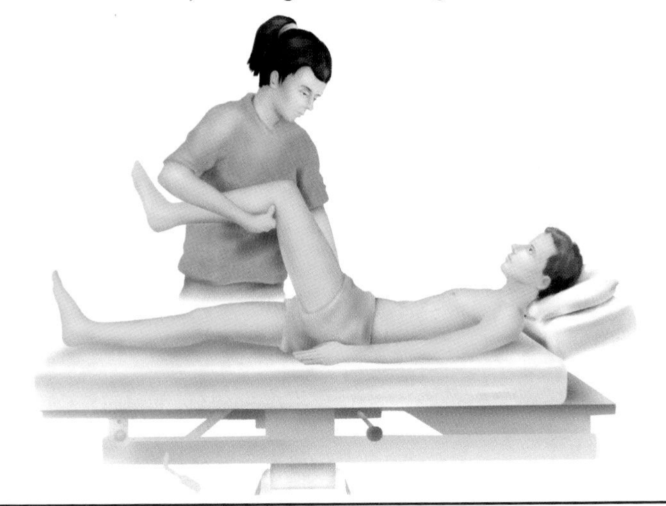

## MANIPULATIVE TECHNIQUES (contd)

- Direct and forceful manipulative techniques which usually involve a high velocity thrust.

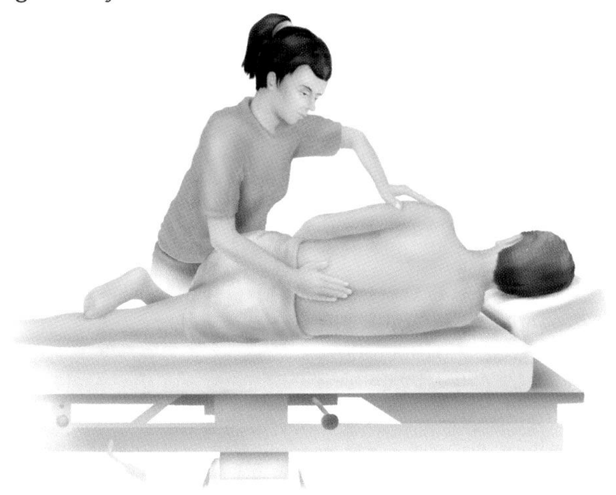

- Cranial osteopathy, which involves gentle and subtle movements that are said to affect the rhythmic pulsation of the fluid around the brain in order to correct problems originating in the nervous system. These usually involve the osteopath holding and gently moving the head.

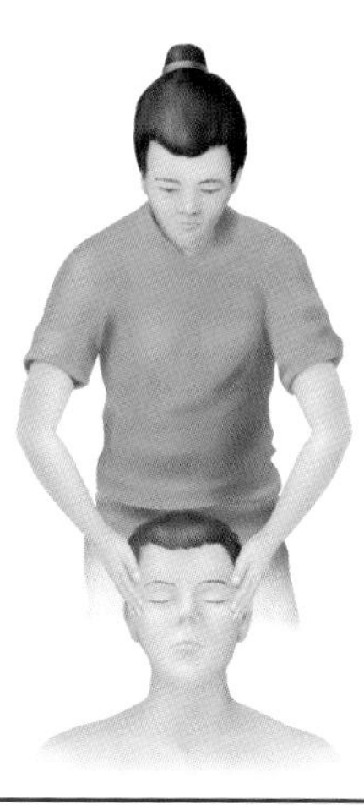

surgical opinion) to an appropriately trained manipulator within six weeks if the pain is persistent. There is considerable research evidence to support this, particularly in relation to chiropractic. Large well-constructed clinical trials suggest that patients receiving manipulation for their back pain are less likely to have a back problem both immediately after the treatment and a year later.

It is unclear whether simple physiotherapy techniques are actually better or worse than manipulation for patients with back and neck pain. As with many other complementary therapies, there is some good scientific evidence that manipulation is of benefit, but these techniques are certainly used far more extensively than would be indicated solely on the basis of the research available.

## How does manipulation work?

The rather fanciful ideas that osteopathy and chiropractic can treat almost anything have now been rejected by the manipulative profession. Manipulators see many of their treatments in the context of a mechanical model. The main aim of these techniques is to restore normal joint movement as quickly as possible. They get rid of pain by improving joint movement and overcoming muscle spasm and any nerve irritation that may be occurring.

Clearly, if a bone is broken, or if a disc is prolapsed and pressing on a nerve, or if there is an active bone infection or inflammation of a joint (for instance, in rheumatoid arthritis), then manipulation is unlikely to be effective and may be harmful.

## What does the treatment involve?

At your first appointment, you need to give a clear history of your problem and the manipulator will examine you carefully. Chiropractors tend to work more swiftly than osteopaths, but usually a first appointment with a manipulator will take between 15 and 45 minutes. The manipulator will need to make a clear diagnosis of whether your problem is musculoskeletal and, if so, which part of that system needs treatment.

You will usually need to get undressed to your underwear so that you can be examined and treated properly. Simple acute back pain usually needs between two and eight sessions. If yours is a chronic, repetitive problem, it may need more treatment.

The essence of good manipulation is a thorough and complete examination. The act of manipulating your spine should occur only after the manipulator has arrived at a proper diagnosis. The diagnosis will sometimes involve taking X-rays and usually involves examining your muscles, bones, joints and nervous system. While the majority of manipulators spend most of their time treating the spine, the peripheral joints, such as knees, hips, elbows and shoulders, can also greatly benefit from these techniques.

Chiropractors tend to suggest that patients come back for preventive adjustments. This means giving you treatments when you are symptom-free every three or six months just to keep you well. Osteopaths may want to see you only when you have symptoms. It is difficult to know which is the best approach, as there is no good evidence upon which to base a choice.

## Is manipulation safe?

Manipulation is one of the areas of complementary medicine where adverse reactions are known to occur. It is vital that you are examined properly and a clear diagnosis made before any manipulation begins.

Manipulation of the neck has been reported to cause stroke and spinal cord injuries, and sometimes these are simply not predictable. Estimates for how frequently these severe reactions occur suggest less than one case per one million manipulations. Temporary adverse reactions are quite common; about a quarter to a half of patients who have had manipulation experience some increased pain or discomfort after the procedure, although the vast majority of these adverse reactions will disappear in 24 hours and are actually part of the treatment process.

There are a number of situations in which manipulation should never be given (contraindications), and these include a fracture, an inflamed joint, a ruptured or unstable ligament in the joint, a mechanically unstable neck, compromised blood circulation in the neck and an inflamed or compressed nerve, either in the spinal canal or coming from the spinal canal. Sometimes, manipulation will need to be carried out very carefully after an operation or in people who have osteoporosis (thinning bones). If you are taking anticoagulants to thin your blood (for example, in heart disease) or you have a very distorted spine, then manipulation would need to be carried out very carefully.

An arthritic joint in itself is not a contraindication to manipulation, and indeed many people who suffer from persistent pain may benefit from treatment. In well-trained hands, manipulation is generally a safe and beneficial procedure.

## WHOM SHOULD I SEE?

Osteopaths and chiropractors are statutorily registered and governed by bodies that can strike them off their register if they fail to comply with proper professional standards and ethics. If the practitioner you wish to see is on the lists provided by either the General Osteopathic Council or the General Chiropractic Council, then you can be assured that they are properly registered and qualified.

Lists of doctors who manipulate can be obtained from the British Institute of Musculoskeletal Medicine. The Manipulation Association of Chartered Physiotherapists will provide information about appropriately qualified physiotherapists. Details of all these bodies can be found in 'Useful addresses' (page 99).

In reality, there may be little to choose from between the manipulative skill and expertise of a physiotherapist and an osteopath or chiropractor and that of a medically qualified orthopaedic physician. What is important is that you feel comfortable with the manipulator whom you see and that their particular approach is of benefit to you.

### KEY POINTS

- ✓ Osteopathy and chiropractic involve a variety of techniques designed to encourage normal movement of muscles, bones and joints
- ✓ These approaches are likely to be helpful in many painful conditions caused by spinal or joint problems
- ✓ Osteopaths and chiropractors should be registered with their professional organisations

# Massage, aromatherapy and reflexology

Therapeutic massage is very much a part of many different traditional medical systems, particularly those originating in Asia. It involves various, usually gentle, manual techniques directed at muscles and connective tissue. It is usually applied to the whole body but can concentrate on specific areas of tenderness or soreness. The aim is to provide general physical relaxation as well as to treat quite specific problems such as neck or low back pain.

The massage techniques that relate to traditional Chinese medicine are almost all centred around the manual stimulation of acupuncture points and the muscles that surround them. This includes techniques such as shiatsu and acupressure.

Traditional European massage techniques were rationalised by Per Hendrik Ling of Sweden, who used vigorous massage of the muscles in the eighteenth century to increase healing and stimulate the circulation of blood and lymph.

Modern Western massage techniques cover a variety of therapies including aromatherapy and reflexology.

In some therapies that involve a 'hands-on' approach, it forms the initial basis through which a physiotherapist may work with your emotional distress.

## Massage techniques

The so-called 'Swedish massage' developed by Per Hendrik Ling has a number of quite specific techniques associated with it (see pages 62 and 63).

## MASSAGE TECHNIQUES

The so-called 'Swedish massage' developed by Per Hendrik Ling has a number of quite specific techniques associated with it. These include:

- *Petrissage,* pressure applied across the width of the muscle

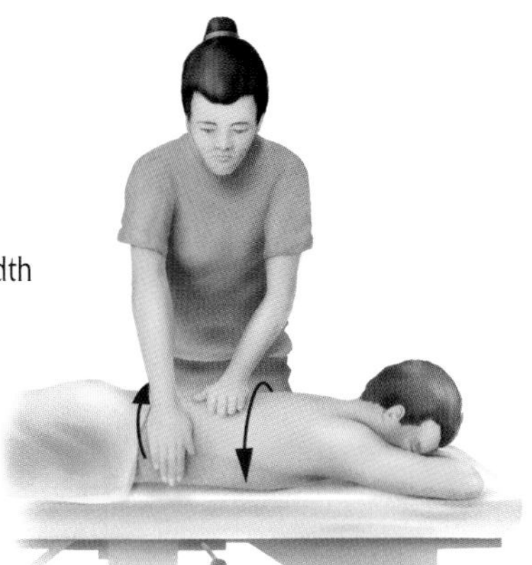

- *Friction,* which is a deep massage applied by circular motions of the thumb or fingertips

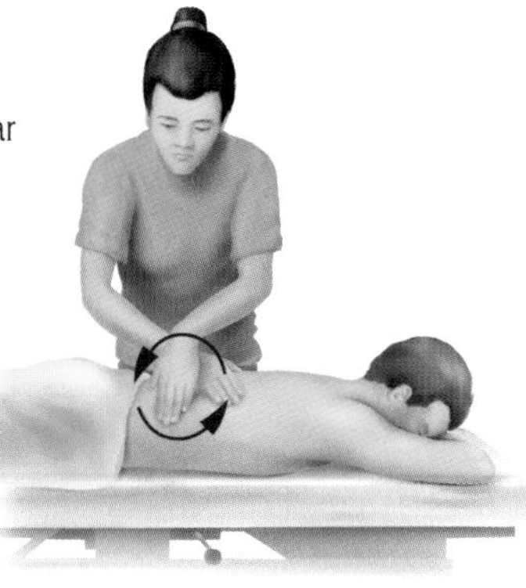

## MASSAGE TECHNIQUES (contd)

- *Effleurage*, gentle stroking along the length of the muscle 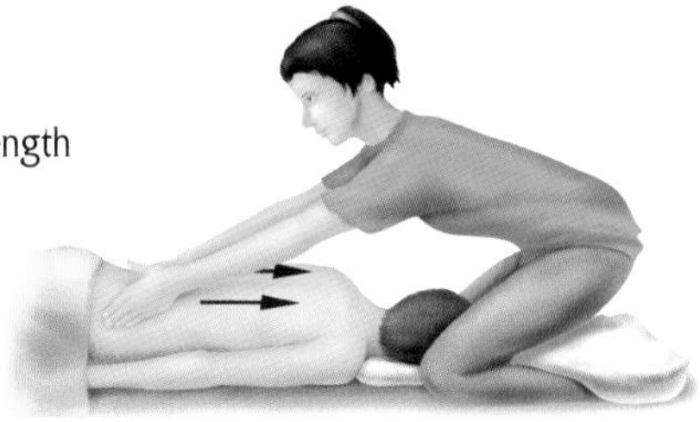
- *Kneading*, which effectively means squeezing the muscle 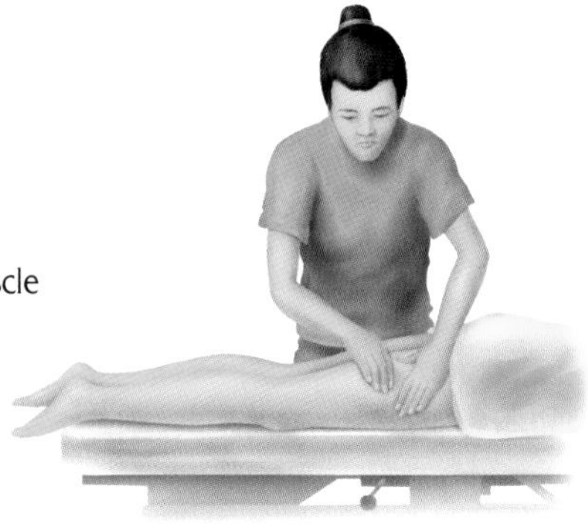
- *Hacking*, involving light slaps or gentle karate chops on the muscle

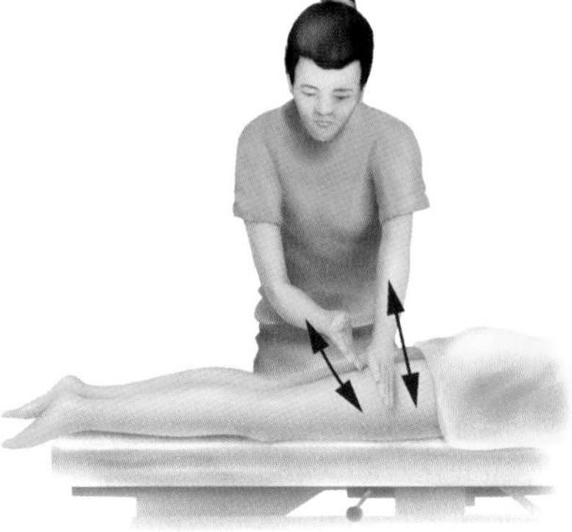

An experienced masseur will use these techniques to heal or improve muscular function, particularly if there has been some injury to a muscle or its attachments.

Some of these techniques, particularly deep friction, are part of conventional physiotherapy. It is difficult to decide whether massage in this context should be considered to be a conventional or complementary medical technique.

Acupressure and shiatsu both involve the treatment of acupuncture points with manual stimulation. A variety of different techniques, which have their origins in acupuncture, are used to treat both acupuncture points and the meridians (energy pathways). The point prescriptions used by therapists will come from both clinical experience and traditional Chinese medicine. It is difficult to decide whether these approaches should be considered as part of acupuncture or part of massage.

## AROMATHERAPY

Aromatherapy involves using essential oils extracted from plants. A French chemist, Monsieur Gattefosse, is said to have burned his hand in a laboratory accident and then plunged it into a vat of lavender oil. He found that the wound healed remarkably quickly without any scarring and coined the term 'aromatherapy' in 1931 to describe this new treatment.

The use of aromas to treat illness appears to have originated with the Australian Aborigines. They had already identified that tea tree oil, an essential oil used in modern aromatherapy, was an excellent antiseptic. The ancient Egyptians used herbal oils for embalming, while their priests used herbs and oils for the treatment of a whole variety of illnesses. Aromatherapy was first publicised in the twentieth century by Dr Valnet, a Frenchman who introduced the use of aromatherapy massage in the 1960s.

Essential oils can be inhaled or may be dropped into a hot bath and absorbed through the skin. Probably the most common use of aromatherapy is to dilute by about one in 10 the essential oil, such as

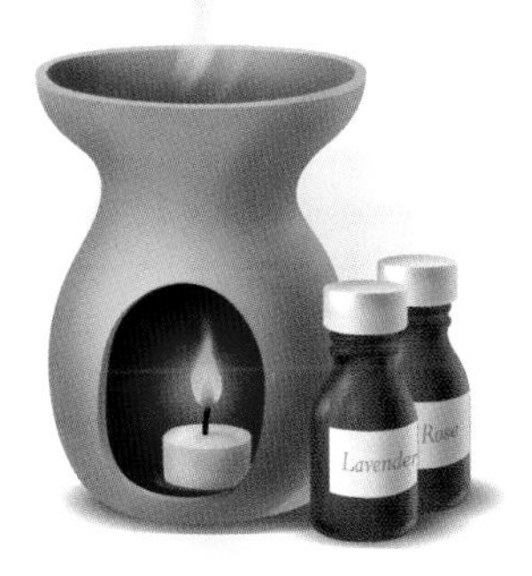

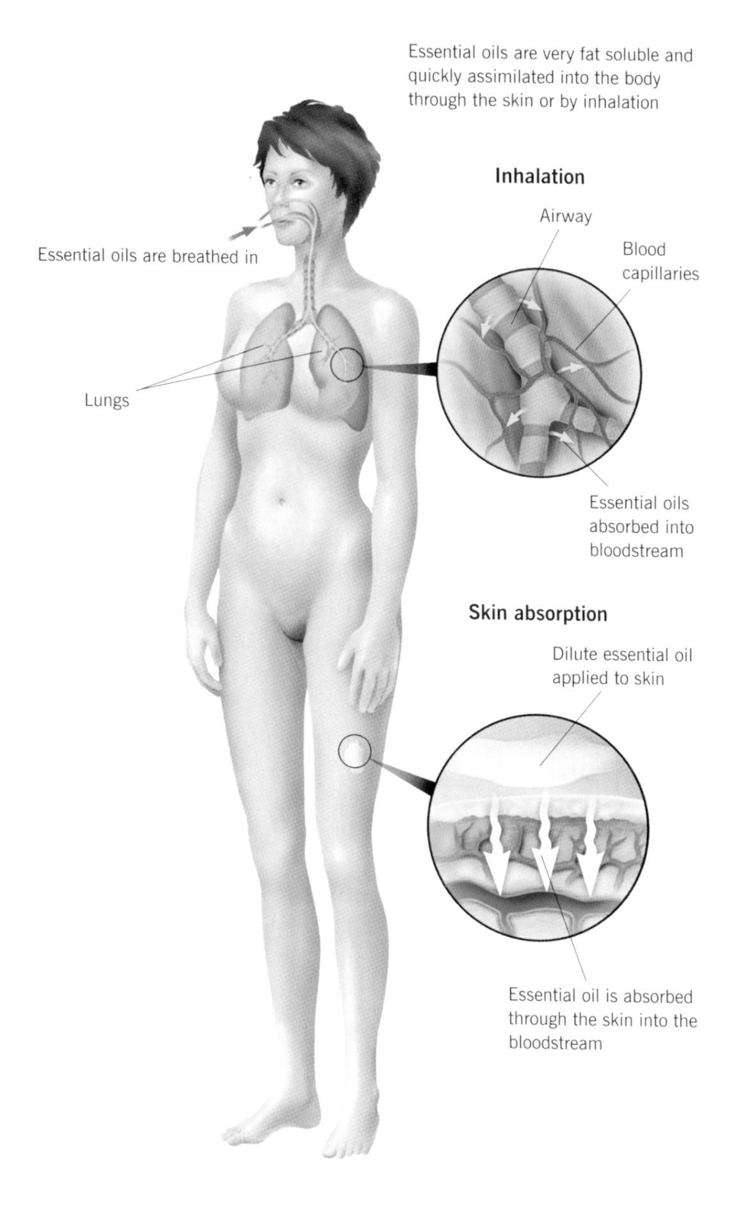


Aromatherapy involves using essential oils extracted from plants. Essential oils can either be inhaled or dropped into a hot bath and absorbed through the skin.

lavender, in a simple vegetable oil base (for example, sweet almond oil) and then use the subsequent mixture for massage – an aromatherapy massage.

The oils themselves are very fat soluble and quickly enter the body either through the skin or by inhalation. Some of the common oils that you may come across include lavender (which is said to help burns and shock, and to aid relaxation and sleep), tea tree oil (which has both anti-bacterial and anti-fungal effects) and neroli (which is said to be particularly useful for anxiety).

Although there has been some research into the specific therapeutic properties claimed for the oils, almost all their usage is based on the clinical experience of practitioners over the last 40 or 50 years.

It is important when using the oils to remember that they should be diluted, because neat oils may damage your skin. If you use the oils for massage, make sure they are diluted by about 90 per cent with a vegetable oil. If you place them in your bath, use only 5 to 10 drops and stay in the bath for no more than 10 minutes.

## Reflexology

Reflexology, or reflex zone therapy as it was originally called, can be applied to almost any area of the body, but it is usually applied to the feet. The feet are said to have various areas that represent the whole structure of the body. This is very similar to some specialist acupuncture techniques. Although there is some good evidence that reflex zones exist in the ear, there is no evidence that they also exist in the feet. Having said this, many reflexologists are able to make surprising diagnoses based on the specific tender areas that exist in the feet.

Although there is much reference to reflex zone therapy in some of the ancient Chinese and Indian texts, modern reflexology was initially developed by Dr William Fitzgerald, an American ear, nose and throat specialist. Fitzgerald mapped the reflex zones on the hands and feet and, in association with Dr Edwin Bowers, published this in 1917. In 1920, another doctor, Joseph Reilly, further developed these techniques and published a book on reflex zone therapy.

Reflexology became popular in the 1960s in the UK through the efforts of Doreen Bailey who met one of Joseph Reilly's assistants and developed the technique.

Reflexology involves applying pressure through the practitioner's hands to the patient's feet, initially for diagnosis. The identification of tender areas can tell the qualified reflexologist which organs might be causing problems. The reflexologist

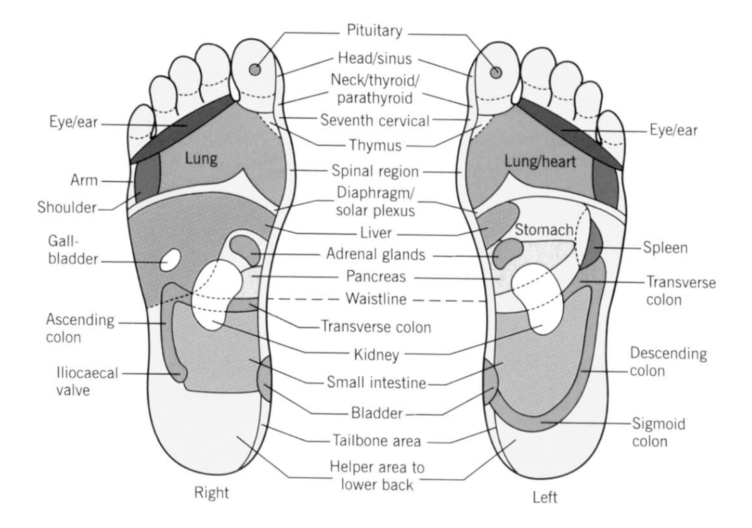


Reflexology can be applied to almost any area of the body, but it is usually applied to the feet. The feet are said to have various zones which represent the whole structure of the body. This is very similar to specialist acupuncture techniques.

will then massage these tender areas on the feet, sometimes causing quite a lot of pain, in order to treat and rebalance any dysfunction. A diagnosis based on reflexology may not be accurate and should never be assumed to correlate directly with a conventional medical diagnosis. You will need both types of diagnostic approach in order to be sure that nothing has been missed.

Reflexology usually involves applying pressure on the bottom, sides and top of the foot and massaging the painful or tender zones deeply with thumb and finger pressure. The treatment itself has a similar range of uses to acupressure, shiatsu and other forms of massage. It can help to induce a general state of relaxation, and can

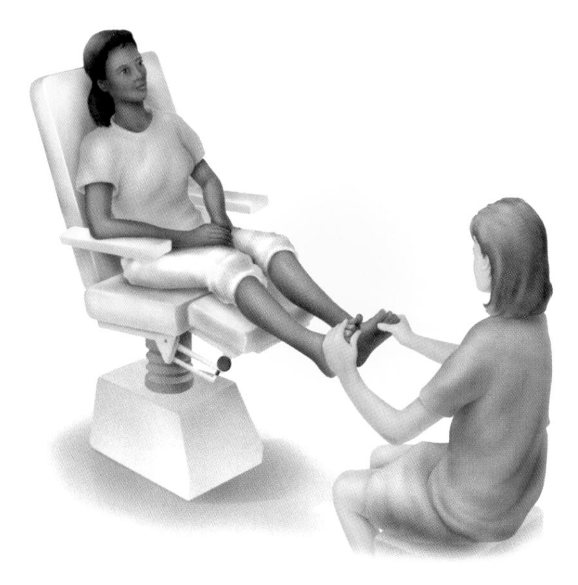

Reflexology involves the practitioner applying pressure with the hands to the patient's feet. The identification of tender areas can tell the qualified reflexologist which organs might be causing problems. The reflexologist will then massage these tender areas on the feet in order to treat and rebalance any dysfunction.

also be of value in the treatment of pain and a number of other conditions.

However, although some therapists believe that reflexology can be of assistance in a wide range of conditions, there is unfortunately very little clinical research within this area. Reflexology treatments are applied on the basis of clinical experience, and it is not realistically possible to recommend reflexology as an effective treatment for any specific condition.

The treatment will usually take about 45 minutes to one hour. If you are going to experience benefit, you will know in the first three or four sessions. The number of treatments you should have, as with all massage therapies, depends on why you went in the first place. Some people like to visit a therapist on a weekly basis just to create their own 'space' and relax, whereas others use it as a maintenance therapy in a chronic illness or to treat pain. Once you know that reflexology is effective for you, it is really up to you and the therapist to decide how many treatments you require.

## What can massage treat?

All massage therapies have powerful relaxing and anti-anxiety effects. This may be partially induced by the actual act of massage, or it may have a much deeper, more comforting effect. For instance, someone who is suffering from terminal cancer may have had some disfiguring operations and could feel very embarrassed about being held or touched by those they love. Massage can offer a physical reassurance for someone's very human needs, and perhaps that is why massage-based therapies are now such a popular part of palliative cancer care. Premature babies who receive regular massage seem to thrive more than their contemporaries who do not have massage.

We are not exactly sure how the various massage therapies work, although we do know that essential oils contain specific and possibly therapeutic chemicals. It is possible that reflexology works in a similar way to acupuncture. However, the actual act of massage in both reflexology and aromatherapy probably shares many of the non-specific mechanisms underlying the general effects of massage therapies.

The scope of these various therapies has not been clearly defined by research. The claims of the various massage therapists would indicate that they all feel that the uses of these particular techniques are very broad. There is no doubt that massage can be an important factor in fostering verbal communication, both in people with emotional problems and in children with disabilities.

Both reflexology, through its zone therapy effect, and aromatherapy, possibly through the chemical effect of some of the oils, claim quite well-defined specific therapeutic effects for various illnesses.

## Is massage therapy safe?

In general, massage therapy is very safe. However, massage should not be used on areas of the body that are damaged, for instance a healing scar or burn. There are no known reasons not to massage people with cancer or those who have had heart attacks.

However, the safety of essential oils is an important issue that is yet to be addressed properly. There is no evidence of any adverse reaction to essential oils other than occasional skin sensitivity, but they are absorbed into the body and have a physiological effect. To date, there is no evidence that these oils can trigger cancer or harm people in any way when they are used correctly. However, essential oils are now being used by people in their own homes and they should be monitored carefully by the professionals using them for any possible long-term adverse reactions. At present, there is no formal reporting system for adverse reactions to essential oils.

Massage-based therapies should not be used diagnostically, as they are not reliable techniques for diagnosing illness.

If you see a massage therapist, you will be in close physical contact with them. This carries some risk, so it is important that you make sure the practitioner is properly registered.

## The practice of massage techniques

Massage techniques are practised in many different environments. Many aromatherapists and reflexologists either practise from their own home or visit your home. Massage techniques are also practised in dedicated complementary medical centres within the NHS, particularly in hospices providing palliative care, as well as in some doctors' surgeries and in environments caring for people with psychological problems.

The practice of these massage techniques should be carried out in a clean and professional environment, whether it is in a hospital or in the community.

## Whom should I contact?

Various organisations provide massage. The Aromatherapy Consortium represents professional registered aromatherapists (see Useful addresses, page 101). There is no specific organisation for reflexologists; the two largest organisations within the reflexology world are the Association of Reflexologists and the International Federation of Reflexologists (pages 105–6).

The massage organisations generally provide both training and registration for their practitioners. Massage skills may be learned by someone who is a qualified nurse or physiotherapist or by someone without any medical background who is simply interested in these techniques. The International Therapy Examination Council (ITEC) holds examinations in massage and related therapies, and it is these examinations that are accepted by most organisations. A practitioner who is a member of one of the proper massage bodies will be regulated and will stick to a proper code of ethics.

## KEY POINTS

- ✓ Massage involves a variety of 'hands-on' techniques designed to relieve stress and improve well-being, as well as treating specific problems
- ✓ Aromatherapy usually involves the use of massage with plant-based oils that have their own effects on the body over and above simple massage
- ✓ Reflexology involves the massage of particular areas on the feet to relieve symptoms or discomfort in other parts of the body
- ✓ All these techniques are safe, but in many instances the effects of these treatments are unproven

# Mind–body therapies, hypnosis and other relaxation techniques

Mind–body medicine recognises the profound connection between the mind and the body, the body's natural healing ability and the role of self-responsibility in the healing process. A wide range of techniques comes under this umbrella, including hypnotherapy, biofeedback, guided imagery, meditation, Qigong, yoga and autogenic training.

The power of suggestion has played a major role in healing for thousands of years. Healing trances have been used by cultures to implant suggestions for self-cure, including the various types of exorcism that were frequently recorded in mediaeval Europe. Over the past 300 years, however, the importance of psychological influences in health and disease has often been neglected.

Franz Anton Mesmer, a Viennese physician, introduced modern hypnotherapy as a method of healing in the late eighteenth century. Mesmer successfully treated a large number of people by inducing deep trances, and explained the healing process with the aid of concepts such as 'stored cosmic fluid' and 'animal magnetism'. However, Mesmer's wild theories and his use of magico-theatrical settings alienated the medical profession, and he was banned from France. *The Lancet* poured scorn on mesmerism: 'We regard its abettors as quacks and imposters.'

James Braid, a Scottish surgeon, in the nineteenth century coined the term 'hypnosis' from *hypnos*, the Greek word for sleep. Despite therapeutically successful demonstrations and Braid's new neurophysiological theories, conventional medical opinion remained hostile

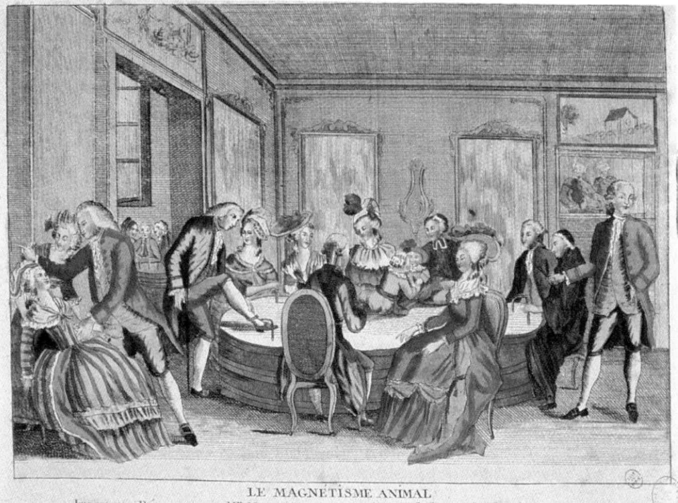


A French engraving of 1784 that shows Franz Anton Mesmer overseeing a demonstration of 'animal magnetism'. Mesmer's wild theories and his use of magico-theatrical settings alienated the medical profession.

until recently to hypnosis, and insisted that the mind could not influence organic disease.

Mind–body techniques encompass a holistic healing philosophy that recognises the remarkable extent to which the mind and nervous system play a role in governing physical and psychological well-being. Chronic stress and unhappiness may contribute to disease, whereas relaxation, positive ways of coping with stress and restoring a more balanced way of life can be used to regain health.

Although mind–body therapies often begin by promoting mental and physical relaxation, they make use of the body's self-healing ability and the person is actively involved in their own treatment. By taking responsibility for their healing, a person's sense of control replaces feelings of helplessness and hopelessness. Mind–body medicine regards illness as a message to the body and looks beyond the immediate problem to review the entire system.

## Hypnotherapy

Hypnosis can be defined as a relaxed state of heightened suggestibility. The state is usually obtained by first relaxing the body, then distracting the conscious mind and heightening the focus of attention on ideas suggested by the therapist or oneself (self-hypnosis). This does not usually involve swinging a pocket watch. It's more like a quiet meditation session.

Modern hypnotherapy does not always involve the stereotypical 'hypnotic trance'. There are various trance states:

- **Light trance (superficial hypnotic state):** The eyes are closed, the person is deeply relaxed and accepts suggestions.

- **Medium trance (fully hypnotised state):** Physiological processes slow down, the person is partially insensible to pain, allergic reactions stop – it is in this state that most therapy is performed.

- **Deep trance (somnambulistic state):** The eyes may be open but total anaesthesia is possible – it is in this state that post-hypnotic suggestions are most successful.

The session usually ends with a few words from the hypnotherapist which bring the patient out of the trance.

Ninety per cent of the population can be hypnotised, with 20 to 30 per cent having enough suggestibility to enter a deep trance, making them highly receptive to treatment.

Conditions essential to successful hypnotherapy include:

- rapport between the therapist and subject

- a comfortable environment, free from distraction

- willingness and cooperation of the subject to participate in the process.

The hypnotic state is used to implant a post-hypnotic suggestion, for example, the desire to stop smoking. The effectiveness of hypnotherapy depends on the extent to which the patient retains the suggestion in their waking state. Suggestions have to be reinforced and maintained by the patient as well as the therapist so self-hypnosis or relaxation is often an important part of the treatment.

A hypnotherapy session may last about one hour. The average number of sessions required to produce results are between 6 and 12, usually once a week. Hypnotherapy can be used for any condition that will benefit from a relaxation technique.

## Biofeedback

Biofeedback training is a process of learning self-regulating abilities. An appropriate monitoring device is used, which enables the person to know when they are controlling a previously 'unconscious' response (such as blood pressure).

The degree to which a person can learn to regulate, consciously, normally unconscious vital functions is quite remarkable. Research has shown that some people can even learn to control brainwave activity, heart rate, skin temperature and gut contraction.

The person is instructed in the use of simple relaxation. This should produce the desired response (for example, lower the blood pressure or body temperature or relax the muscles), and an electronic device is used to provide feedback to see whether the relaxation is achieving the desired effect. The feedback used in the technique should be designed to suit the individual and help him or her to relax.

The courses of treatment vary in length, with most being 10 to 15 half-hour weekly sessions. Biofeedback skills appear to improve with daily practice.

## Guided imagery or visualisation

Guided imagery is a process that involves using the conscious mind to create mental images to evoke physical changes, promote natural healing and provide insight and self-awareness. Imagery in a relaxed state of mind is a component of most of the mind–body techniques and can be achieved through use of images suggested by the therapist.

The first reported visualisation techniques in the mid-1970s used aggressive images such as sharks attacking and killing cancer cells. However, while these may be helpful to some people, they may induce negative feelings in others. Nowadays, more positive images are used – relaxation, cancer cells being carried out of the body, pain being controlled with calmness and serenity.

## Meditation

Meditation can be broadly defined as any activity that keeps the mind calm and pleasantly focused in the present moment, so that it is neither reacting to memories from the past, nor being preoccupied with plans for the future.

Although meditation covers a wide range of techniques, these can be grouped into two basic approaches:

- Concentrative meditation involves focusing the attention on breathing, an image or a sound ('mantra'), so that the mind becomes more tranquil and aware.

- Mindfulness meditation involves opening the attention to whatever goes through the mind, without thoughts or worries, so that the mind becomes calm and clear.

A number of studies have shown that the state of deep relaxation produced by meditation is accompanied by various physiological and biochemical changes, including decreased heart rate, blood pressure, respiratory rate, muscle tone and electrical skin conduction, and increased brainwaves. Mindfulness meditation has been thoroughly researched as an effective way of treating anxiety, chronic pain and panic disorder.

## Qigong

Qigong is the practice of activating, refining and circulating the human 'energy field'. Qigong literally means 'energy cultivation' and is a cornerstone of traditional Chinese medicine. It is perhaps the oldest known method of physical, mental, emotional and spiritual healing, and combines slow graceful movements with imagery, mental concentration, sounds that affect body organs and breathing control to increase a person's 'life force'. The three key elements of Qigong are:

- regulating the body through postures and movements
- regulating breathing using breathing control exercises
- regulating the mind through mental focusing and visualisation methods.

## Yoga

Yoga originated in India and provides a complete system of physical, mental and spiritual health. Yoga means 'union', and physical postures, breathing exercises and meditation practices are used to achieve mind–body–spirit unity.

Classical yoga is organised into eight 'limbs', which include lifestyle, hygiene and detoxification regimens, together with physical and psychological practices. The first four limbs consist of postures from breathing exercises that serve to bring the mind and body into harmony. The remaining four limbs involve meditative practices. Yoga postures are designed to create a condition of ease in the body to facilitate meditation, or may be applied therapeutically for specific physical disorders.

Breathing control, or 'pranayama', exercises are designed to promote the free and even flow of prana ('life force') throughout the body. Pranayama can help to regulate the previously unconscious bodily function, and to promote a calm and focused state of mind in preparation for meditation.

Samadhi ('spiritual realisation') is the final stage of yoga and can be achieved only through long-disciplined and dedicated practice. A person is said to enter a fourth state of consciousness, separate

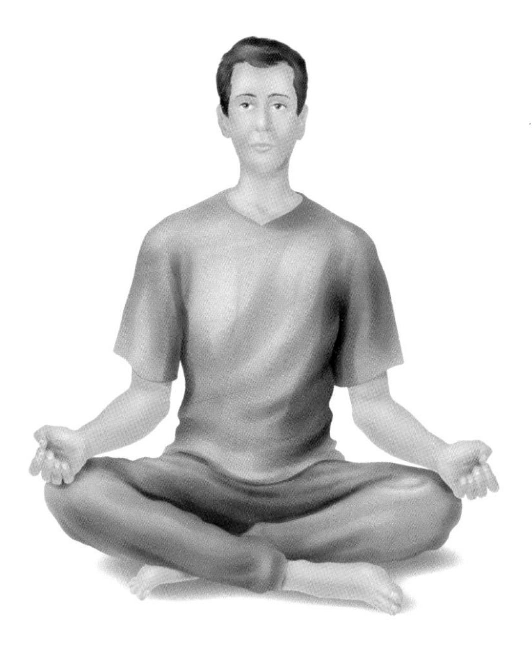

Yoga originated in India and provides a complete system of physical, mental and spiritual health. Physical postures, breathing exercises and meditation are used to achieve mind–body–spirit unity.

from and beyond the ordinary states of waking, dreaming and sleep.

## AUTOGENIC THERAPY

Autogenic therapy is a self-help method that produces profound relaxation and relief from the negative effects of stress. 'Autogenic' means 'generated from within'.

The standard autogenic formulae were originated by Dr Johannes Schultz in the 1920s in Berlin. Autogenic therapy (often known as autogenic training) was further developed in Canada by his colleague Dr Wolfgang Luthe. It is taught in many countries, especially in continental Europe and Canada. It was introduced to Britain in the 1970s and the British Association for Autogenic Training and Therapy (BAFATT) was formed in 1984. BAFATT is a registered charity founded for the purpose of training therapists and maintaining professional standards.

The technique mobilises our natural systems for healing and

recuperation. It consists of a series of simple, easily learned mental exercises that link mind and body together in association with deep relaxation. These exercises enable the mind to calm itself by switching off the body's stress responses.

The standard autogenic exercises can be adapted to include personal motivational formulae, affirmations or healing formulae. In addition, various additional mental exercises can be introduced – some to help deal with the lingering effects of past experience and others to allow calming in a stressful situation.

## What can mind–body therapies be used for?

Beyond simple relaxation, mind–body therapies have a wide range of uses. Because these methods treat the whole person rather than symptoms or diseases, they can be applied to almost any health problem. In addition, in healthy people, mind–body techniques (particularly Qigong, yoga and meditation) may be useful in health maintenance, disease prevention, the enhancement of well-being and spiritual growth.

Scientific studies have evaluated a number of these mind–body therapies.

Hypnotherapy has been used to treat pain, irritable bowel syndrome and asthma effectively, and appears to be as good as any other approaches to smoking cessation.

Biofeedback has been shown to be of value in migraine, tension headaches, raised blood pressure and urinary incontinence.

Guided imagery is certainly an easy way to relax and, although there are few clinical trials, it has been used in a wide range of conditions including pain, asthma, raised blood pressure and irritable bowel syndrome as well as in the treatment of AIDS and cancer.

Meditation has been used to treat anxiety and depression in cancer patients as well as stress and pain.

There are very few good quality clinical trials evaluating Qigong, but a wide range of studies have been used to evaluate and understand autogenic therapy and do show that it is beneficial for many people.

## How do these therapies work?

Mind–body therapies support and encourage the body's internal healing mechanism. Our understanding of healing and how the mind can affect the immune system (psychoneuroimmunology) has increased dramatically over the last two decades. We now understand that various chemicals released during relaxed emotional states enhance healing and relax the automatic or unconscious part of the nervous system so that it becomes less 'stressed and tense'. These psychoneuroimmunological effects do have a direct positive effect on our immune status and the activity of our white blood cells.

## Is it safe?

These methods are generally very safe, and there are few precautions or side effects provided that they are competently taught and appropriately applied. As with any form of treatment it is, of course, essential that a proper diagnosis is made first, and the limitations of the method recognised. Hypnosis should not be performed on patients with psychosis, organic psychiatric conditions or antisocial personality disorders because the hypnotic process may strengthen their condition.

## Who should I consult?

There are various different organisations for each of the therapies. In the case of doctors practising any of these techniques, the General Medical Council regulates the ethical and professional standards of medical behaviour. Psychologists practising these therapies are certified and registered by the British Psychological Society. Practitioners who are neither doctors nor psychologists are regulated mainly by their professional training and therapy organisations.

## KEY POINTS

- ✓ Mind–body therapies involve various techniques and states of mind designed to promote well-being and relaxation
- ✓ These approaches can be of benefit in helping people cope with and manage many chronic illnesses

# Nutritional medicine

Nutritional medicine involves modifying a person's diet as well as recommending or prescribing vitamin and mineral supplements, usually taken by mouth, in the form of tablets or liquids. For any living organism to function properly, a number of vitamins (usually described by the letters A to E) and minerals (such as zinc, magnesium and chromium) are essential.

Their absence leads to disease, an observation first noted by James Lind in 1753. He was a naval doctor who observed that sailors on long voyages who had no access to fresh fruit and vegetables developed scurvy. This deficiency disease could kill a significant proportion of the crew, consequently reducing the navy's ability to fight or man their ships. Lind observed that the addition of lime juice to the sailors' diet could prevent scurvy. Vitamin C itself, however, was not chemically isolated until the twentieth century. A whole series of specific diseases, such as pellagra and beri-beri (both deficiency diseases of the vitamin B group), were carefully documented, and their cause isolated, in the 1920s and 1930s.

The dietary recommendations made by most Western governments tend to be more focused on avoiding deficiencies rather than promoting optimal health. Most experts are sure about the nutritional requirements that are needed to avoid illness. However, there is often little information, and indeed much argument in the nutritional world, about the doses of nutritional supplements required to sustain optimal health. This is particularly so for the needs of people whose nutritional demands are raised for some reason, such as the presence of disease or when subject to unusual physical or mental demands, such as competitive sport.

This is perhaps illustrated by the differences in reference nutrient intakes (RNIs) between the USA and the UK – nearly all the RNIs in the USA are higher than those in the UK even though the Government has recently increased its recommended RNI for the UK population.

The table on page 82 shows the RNIs for some common vitamins and minerals and also shows how much of the average UK population falls below the recommended intakes. This suggests a somewhat worrying picture. Although many people in the UK certainly eat enough to suffer from obesity, a significant minority is probably also suffering from nutritional deficiencies. This is probably associated with the rise of high-fat, high-carbohydrate and low-nutrient junk food, as well as the increase in industrialised farming, which produces products with relatively lower levels of vitamins and minerals.

## Is nutritional medicine conventional or complementary?

The various vitamins and minerals are a very important part of conventional medicine. However, many conventional doctors just assume that the average British diet is nutritionally adequate and other than in specific illnesses, such as eating disorders or anaemia, will rarely investigate a person's nutritional status. There are some types of nutritional medicine, generally described as orthomolecular medicine, in which very large doses of vitamins and minerals are used to treat illnesses varying from the common cold to cancer.

One of the underlying principles of nutritional medicine is that each person is unique and has unique nutritional requirements, so that what may be an adequate nutritional intake for one person may be inappropriate for another.

## What should nutritional medicine be used for?

Nutritional medicine has a range of uses spanning both conventional and complementary medicine. Some nutritional experts argue that everyone needs to take regular nutritional supplements on a daily basis, whereas others suggest that nutritional supplements are needed only where there is a proven deficiency, such as in iron-deficiency anaemia.

Certainly, nutritional supplements can be effectively used to modify the way some illnesses affect us. For example, there is

## PERCENTAGE OF UK MEN AND WOMEN (19–50 YEARS) WITH DIETARY INTAKES OF VITAMINS AND MINERALS BELOW THE REFERENCE NUTRIENT INTAKE (RNI)

| Nutrient | RNI | | Less than RNI (%) | |
|---|---|---|---|---|
| | Men | Women | Men | Women |
| **VITAMINS** | | | | |
| Vitamin A | 700 μg | 600 μg | 27% | 31% |
| Riboflavin | 1.3 mg | 1.1 mg | 12% | 21% |
| Pyridoxine | 1.4 mg | 1.2 mg | 6% | 22% |
| Vitamin $B_{12}$ | 1.5 μg | 1.5 μg | 1% | 4% |
| Folate | 200 μg | 200 μg | 12% | 47% |
| Vitamin C | 40 mg | 40 mg | 26% | 34% |
| **MINERALS** | | | | |
| Calcium | 700 mg | 700 mg | 25% | 48% |
| Magnesium | 300 mg | 300 mg | 42% | 72% |
| Iron | 8.7 mg | 14.8 mg | 12% | 89% |
| Zinc | 9.5 mg | 7 mg | 31% | 31% |
| Copper | 1.2 mg | 1.2 mg | 24% | 59% |
| Iodine | 140 μg | 140 μg | 9% | 32% |
| Potassium | 3,500 mg | 3,500 mg | 65% | 94% |

Source: MAFF 1994 – *The Dietary and Nutritional Survey of British Adults.*

**Key**
RNI = reference nutrient intake
μg = micrograms (one-millionth part of a gram)
mg = milligrams (one-thousandth part of a gram)

evidence that zinc taken orally will shorten the duration of a cold or flu and alleviate the symptoms. Eating more polyunsaturated fatty acids, usually derived from plants or, more commonly, fish oils, can reduce the levels of harmful fats in the blood, control and reduce inflammation in rheumatoid arthritis and even ease symptoms and reduce relapse rates in inflammatory bowel disease (such as ulcerative colitis and Crohn's disease).

Studies suggest that vitamin C probably does treat (although it does not prevent) colds, vitamin $B_6$ is of value in premenstrual syndrome and possibly autism, while vitamin E may be of value for people with angina. It is known that folic acid, taken before and during pregnancy, will reduce the rate of spina bifida (a neural tube defect) in babies. In general, the intake of folic acid in most Westernised industrialised nations falls well below the recommended nutritional intake – one American study suggested that most adults were taking only half the RNI for folate as part of their regular daily diet. Nutritional medicine, therefore, can be very important in the treatment and prevention of various problems.

The recommendations made by some nutritional medicine practitioners frequently involve quite complex and expensive supplement regimens. Many people claim that these regimens are beneficial and, indeed, these may be of genuine benefit. However, medical experts are often unclear about the scientific validity of the very specific recommendations made by some practitioners.

## WHO PRESCRIBES SUPPLEMENTS?

Most people taking nutritional supplements do so on the advice of health magazines, friends or perhaps someone in a health food store or pharmacy selling nutritional supplements. Many people take cod liver oil or glucosamine for their arthritis, and women frequently take extra calcium during and after the menopause to avoid osteoporosis. In other words, most nutritional supplements are taken because people have prescribed them for themselves.

Nutritional supplements may also be used as part of the treatment regimens prescribed by many complementary practitioners, including herbalists, homeopaths, osteopaths and chiropractors. Some therapists specialise in the investigation and prescription of nutritional supplements, in particular those who are members of the British Association of Nutritional Therapists, registered naturopaths and medically qualified doctors who are members of the British Society for Allergy, Environmental and Nutritional Medicine (BSAENM).

## WHAT DOES TREATMENT INVOLVE?

Although, in most cases, nutritional prescriptions are based on a detailed history from the patient, practitioners may use various individual nutritional tests to understand the person's requirements. Sometimes these tests are unconventional and unproven. The more conventional testing methods may be done on blood, hair or sweat and provide a clear and reproducible understanding of whether a person's nutritional status, with respect to the substances being tested, is within the normal range.

The laboratory that conducts most of these nutritional tests in the UK is called Biolab. Biolab will accept requests for tests made by someone who is properly qualified, but does not run investigations requested by members of the general public.

Using these various nutritional investigations enables a properly qualified person to then recommend a specific range of supplements and appropriate dietary changes. Treatments may be designed either to prevent illness or to treat and manage an ongoing complaint.

## Is it safe?

There has recently been a lot of discussion about the safety of nutritional supplements. There is no doubt that some supplements taken in high doses can produce adverse reactions. For example, extra vitamin A is not recommended in pregnancy because it may cause abnormalities in the developing baby. High doses of vitamin C can cause diarrhoea.

In general terms, nutritional supplements taken for two or three months are very unlikely to cause adverse reactions. However, some supplements taken over a long period of time can be harmful. For example, vitamin $B_6$ taken for premenstrual syndrome has, in a very small number of cases, been reported to cause nerve damage. This has usually involved very high doses, far higher than those usually recommended by responsible nutritional therapists. Excessive doses of zinc and selenium have been reported in some cases to suppress the immune system and the prolonged use of evening primrose oil may make some forms of epilepsy slightly worse.

However, it is important to stress that, in general, nutritional supplements are very safe. There have, for example, been no reported deaths due to nutritional supplementation in the UK.

## Whom should I see?

Members of the British Society for Allergy, Environmental and Nutritional Medicine are all medically qualified doctors. The organisation can provide names and addresses of doctors giving nutritional advice and support. The regulation of doctors is the responsibility of the General Medical Council.

The General Council and Register of Naturopaths and the British Association of Nutritional Therapists are educational and regulatory bodies primarily for non-medically qualified people. Details may be found in 'Useful addresses' on page 104.

## KEY POINTS

- ✓ Many people have diets that are poor in essential nutrients
- ✓ Specific nutritional tests are available at specialised laboratories
- ✓ Specific diets and nutritional supplements may be of value in treating illness and maintaining health

# Therapeutic diets

All systems of medicine use diet in one form or another. Conventional doctors are concerned about patients both being overweight and underweight, as well as the quality and type of food that forms part of the modern diet. There are, however, a number of diets that are part of a complementary medical approach.

## Diets as part of treatment

A traditional Chinese doctor may not only recommend acupuncture and various herbs, but also a specific dietary regimen tailored to the individual's constitution. Other complementary therapies, including naturopathy (see page 90), use fasts to clear out 'toxins' before beginning a more specific treatment regimen.

## Disease-specific diets

Particular diets to treat arthritis are not uncommon – for example, avoiding 'acidic' foods such as tomatoes and citrus fruits or introducing specific foods such as cider vinegar. People with catarrh or other chesty symptoms are often given milk-exclusion or milk-free diets to decrease mucus secretion.

## Food-avoidance diets

These diets are suggested to treat a specific illness. Childhood eczema or irritable bowel syndrome may sometimes be managed by an individually tailored diet. Specific-food avoidance regimens are a controversial area and one in which there may be conflict between conventionally trained and medically qualified allergists and CAM practitioners.

## Allergy and intolerance

Food allergy is a very clear and unpleasant reaction to food. For example, if somebody is allergic to shrimps or peanuts they will, within a fairly short time of eating them (usually minutes), experience an immediate allergic reaction. This reaction may give rise to unpleasant swellings in the face or throat and, sometimes, acute asthma. Usually these reactions pass within 20 or 30 minutes and can be treated with anti-allergic drugs such as antihistamines. Sometimes, however, they can be potentially life threatening because they progress to anaphylactic shock. Anaphylaxis is a very acute allergic reaction in which the throat and breathing tube become so swollen that they close up for a short period of time. Anaphylaxis is completely reversible with an injection of adrenaline.

Food allergy is usually quite straightforward to diagnose using blood and skin tests. Once the culprit food or foods have been identified, the person concerned must avoid them completely for the rest of their life. If you have a true food allergy, you must seek the advice of a conventional allergist and carry an adrenaline injection with you at all times in case you unknowingly eat the food to which you are allergic.

Food intolerance works through different mechanisms from allergy, although these mechanisms have not yet been clearly defined. From a medical standpoint, various conditions will improve with long-term food avoidance. These include migraine, arthritis, inappropriate or hyperactive behaviour among children, childhood eczema, irritable bowel syndrome and inflammatory bowel disease, such as colitis and Crohn's disease. All of these conditions have been shown to have a dietary link. There is no particular food for any specific condition – each individual will need to follow their own unique diet to improve their condition.

Although the mechanism of food intolerance is unknown, it is clear that people with these conditions may be 'addicted' to the food to which they are intolerant. For example, a child with eczema may be eating mainly milk, yoghurt and cheese, and it may be milk that is aggravating or causing his or her eczema. Food addiction often runs side by side with food intolerance.

Food intolerance is masked. This means that until the susceptible person has avoided the food, often for three or four weeks, there may be no improvement in their symptoms. While the phenomenon of food intolerance is well documented, and there are a number of studies demonstrating the benefit of avoiding 'culprit' foods, there is no completely reliable method for diagnosing food intolerance.

- Putting people on diets that are unlikely to contain triggers for allergy or food intolerance is the simplest diagnostic process but takes a long time. For instance, a 'stone age' diet of fruit, meat and a few vegetables will often clear the symptoms over a three- or four-week period. Other foods then need to be reintroduced very slowly and the person's acute reaction carefully monitored over a month or two to identify the foods to which they are intolerant.

- Various unconventional tests have been used to work out 'safe' and 'unsafe' foods on an individual basis. Some involve unconventional blood tests in which food extracts are placed in a small tube along with red and white blood cells, and the reaction of the blood cells is monitored microscopically. None of these tests is completely reliable and none has been satisfactorily scientifically validated. However, both practitioners and patients may find some of these tests useful in sorting out their food intolerances while we await further research.

## Do diets produce benefit?

Eating less 'junk food' would certainly benefit the health of both adults and children. There is also clear evidence that specific food-avoidance diets can help with certain conditions.

The use of dietary intervention in childhood behavioural problems has been discussed in the medical literature for the last 45 years and, although diets are not the only way of managing this condition, the evidence that they may be effective in a significant proportion of children is impressive. People with bowel inflammation have fewer relapses if they avoid the specific foods that upset them.

Although medical experts know that food intolerance does have an effect on some illnesses, there is much confusion about how the principles should be applied by doctors when treating their patients. This is partly because there is no clear explanation for how dietary changes might be working and because of the very unconventional and unreliable nature of the tests that are employed to 'unmask' food intolerance.

## What does treatment involve?

Before embarking on a long-term

diet that you have read about in a book, seek advice from your GP, a relevant specialist or a dietitian. What is likely to happen in a consultation about your diet will, to some extent, depend on the methods used to try to isolate your food intolerance. If this is primarily based on dietary avoidance and food reintroduction then you may need several consultations and it will be quite a long process. If one of the unconventional diagnostic methods is used, the diagnostic process may be quite short and you may simply be asked to follow a specific diet for four to six weeks before returning to discuss your symptoms.

You should never be left on a long-term diet without a follow-up appointment within one to two months. Diets should always be used as part of your overall management plan and you should always be supported with appropriate nutritional advice. This will ensure that any diet you use in the long term to control your symptoms does not result in any vitamin or mineral deficiencies a year or two later.

## Is dietary avoidance safe?

In general, and in responsible hands, dietary treatment is a particularly safe approach to illness. Such diets are also very empowering in that you can begin to control your own illness through the foods that you eat.

There are two major potential problems, however, with using food avoidance diets in the long term. The first is the possible risk of developing nutritional deficiencies – this can be avoided with appropriate follow-up appointments and sound nutritional advice.

The second is that long-term diets can be psychologically damaging and can, in effect, become part of a more generalised eating disorder. For example, telling an obsessional young woman to avoid milk or wheat on a long-term basis may actually fuel a pre-existing tendency for her to develop an eating disorder. Diets therefore need to be used in a responsible and conscientious manner.

## Whom should I see?

Nutritional advice is provided by a wide range of complementary and conventional medical practitioners. The British Society for Allergy, Environmental and Nutritional Medicine is open only to doctors, and their members provide advice about both nutritional supplements and food avoidance diets.

Dietitians are qualified registered individuals who work with doctors within the NHS and can provide advice about nutritionally adequate diets, although in general they have limited expertise about food intolerance and food avoidance. Your can contact a dietitian through the British Dietetic Association. Details of these organisations can be found in 'Useful addresses' on page 104.

Naturopaths, who use a therapeutic system based on the concept of 'nature cure', almost invariably incorporate dietary intervention into their practice as well as exercise, homeopathy, herbal medicine and often some acupuncture as well. There are a relatively small number of naturopaths in the UK – it is a much more popular speciality in certain parts of the USA. To find a naturopath in your area, contact the General Council and Register of Naturopaths.

The British Association of Nutritional Therapists encompasses complementary practitioners who are not medically qualified, but are trained in nutritional medicine, and who recommend a wide variety of different nutritional and dietary approaches.

## KEY POINTS

- ✓ There is some evidence that specific-food avoidance diets will help with some chronic complaints such as headache and irritable bowel syndrome
- ✓ There are no reliable tests for food intolerance
- ✓ Food allergy and food intolerance describe different reactions to normal foods
- ✓ Food-avoidance diets are generally safe, provided that they are properly monitored and vitamin and mineral supplements are taken where needed

# Who provides complementary therapies?

Complementary medicine is provided by two groups of therapists. The first are those who have had a formal medical training as doctors, nurses or physiotherapists. The second have had no conventional medical training but have instead been trained in complementary alternative medicine (CAM) disciplines as, for example, osteopaths, chiropractors, professional acupuncturists, medical herbalists and non-medically qualified homeopaths.

It is difficult to say exactly how many complementary medical practitioners there are in the UK. Current estimates from the relevant societies suggest that in 1997 there were 40,000 practitioners with three disciplines representing over half of the registered individuals; healers accounted for 14,000 practitioners, and there were 7,000 aromatherapists and 5,000 reflexologists.

If we look at the therapies that most people seem to use, these include acupuncture, homeopathy, herbal medicine and manipulative medicine (osteopathy and chiropractic). Those practising full-time, such as chiropractors and osteopaths, may be fewer in number but, in comparison to a part-time reflexologist, may treat a far larger number of people. This makes a therapy like chiropractic a far more popular and available choice, even though there are only 1,000 registered chiropractors and 1,000 registered osteopaths in the UK.

Only two groups of CAM practitioners have achieved statutory regulation: osteopaths and chiropractors. Statutory regulation means that these professions have a legally constituted council similar to that for doctors and nurses and someone can call him- or herself an osteopath or a chiropractor only if he or she is trained and registered.

Medical herbalists, acupuncturists and non-medically qualified homeopaths are regulated by voluntary bodies, but are moving towards statutory regulation with the support of the Department of Health. Most of the other CAM professions are voluntarily or self-regulated and you should be very suspicious of a CAM practitioner who is not part of some self-regulatory organisation.

## Medically qualified practitioners

The main CAM therapies provided by doctors are homeopathy, hypnotherapy and acupuncture. The British Medical Acupuncture Society has roughly 2,000 members, most of whom are doctors, although a small number of vets and dentists are also members. Most medically qualified acupuncturists provide an acupuncture service as part of their day-to-day NHS commitment in either hospital or general practice, although many medical acupuncturists also have a small private clinic. The greatest use of acupuncture in hospitals is focused on rheumatology and pain clinics, where acupuncture is used primarily with conventional medicine to treat persistent pain, sometimes with a Western acupuncture approach and sometimes on a traditional Chinese medicine basis. In general practice, acupuncture is also largely used to treat pain and headaches.

The Faculty of Homeopathy represents the medically registered homeopaths. In order to become a Member or Fellow of the Faculty, doctors must pass a very stringent specialist examination in homeopathy. As it is so difficult, and because there is such a limited career structure within medical homeopathy in the UK, there are only just over 200 medically qualified specialist homeopaths. However, this does not represent the extent of clinical practice within medical homeopathy. For example, one of the most popular medical postgraduate courses in Scotland is run by the Glasgow Homeopathic Hospital introducing the use of simple homeopathic techniques into primary care; 20 per cent of Scotland's GPs have attended these basic courses.

The most common complementary therapy provided by physiotherapists is acupuncture. It is now a recognised part of physiotherapy practice and approximately 15 per cent of physiotherapists have an acupuncture qualification. Some physiotherapists and doctors use Western acupuncture techniques, whereas others use techniques firmly grounded in traditional Chinese medicine. Some physiotherapists also use manipulative medicine, and in many cases are experienced in techniques that are very similar, if not the same, as those used by osteopaths and chiropractors.

It is difficult to estimate how many nurses practise CAM, but the CAM special interest group is the largest in the Royal College of Nursing. In general, nurses have focused their interest on massage and therapies such as therapeutic touch, aromatherapy and reflexology.

## Non-medically qualified practitioners

These practitioners come from a complementary medical background and have no conventional medical training. They include osteopaths, chiropractors, professional acupuncturists, medical herbalists and non-medically qualified homeopaths.

Many complementary practitioners have become increasingly interested in obtaining statutory regulation. Osteopaths and chiropractors have the same kind of legally established regulatory body as all the other medical professions. At the moment, they are still thought of as complementary medical practitioners, but in reality they have become part of the medical establishment in the UK. Herbalists and acupuncturists, both of whom complete detailed full-time three- or four-year courses, may soon also begin the process of statutory regulation.

Almost all CAM has some form of organisation and self-regulation. This, as a minimum, includes basic training requirements to ensure that practitioners are safe and competent. They need to understand when the therapy should be applied, and also when it is not suitable and when patients should see another practitioner or their own GP.

Most therapy organisations have clear ethical guidelines, so that the patient's confidentiality is protected, and all practitioners who use patients' personal details on computer should fulfil the requirements of the Data Protection Act. Research supported by the Department of Health and carried out by the University of Exeter has discovered that most complementary medical organisations are following these general guidelines.

It would certainly be wise for anyone thinking of having a CAM treatment to consider whether the therapist is competent, and whether the therapy itself can be provided in a proper and professional manner. Ideally, you should discuss this with your own

GP and the complementary therapist you are thinking of consulting. If you are unsure or concerned about any of these issues, ask again and do not see a practitioner until you are happy that he or she is safe and competent.

## Where is CAM provided?

Most CAM practitioners work on their own, either in their homes or in their own practices. Increasingly, complementary medical centres are developing in the high streets, but in most cases these are simply environments in which various CAM practitioners work, usually by renting rooms. There is also no real integration, either between individual CAM practitioners or between the local medical services and the complementary medical centres. Although many CAM practitioners are particularly skilled within their own professions, this lack of integration is not always good for the patient, who may possibly benefit from a package of treatment (for example, dietary advice, nutritional supplements and manipulation for back pain).

## How can I be referred to a complementary practitioner?

Many people are recommended to a practitioner by a friend or someone who has been successfully treated. They may think that their own doctors may be reluctant to refer them, but information about the behaviour of GPs shows that this belief is false. Referral from the GP is a common route to CAM treatment. In the mid-1980s, around 75 per cent of GPs in some areas of the UK were regularly suggesting that patients see CAM practitioners, based largely on their own personal experiences of the effectiveness of these therapies. They were particularly supportive of making referrals to osteopaths and chiropractors for back pain.

Over the last 15 years, the availability of CAM within the NHS has increased. A survey in the mid-1990s indicated that 40 per cent of general practices were offering some form of CAM therapy. Some was given by the doctors themselves or practice nurses, some by employed CAM practitioners and some by CAM practitioners who rented rooms in the health centres for the convenience of patients.

It is often very difficult for a GP to know to whom to refer and for what. This is partly because most GPs have very little training, knowledge or experience of CAM. This is now changing as more medical schools run CAM familiarisation courses as part of their undergraduate curriculum. It is also because there is so little information as to how to use CAM effectively in any particular situation.

Referral to an acupuncturist for pain or to a manipulator for a bad back is simple and straightforward. Other referrals, say to a herbalist or a homeopath, may need some discussion between you and your doctor, along with some information that you or the relevant therapy organisation may provide such as when it may be appropriate to seek their advice. It is impossible to lay down absolute guidelines for when such referrals should take place, but in general both you and your GP may wish to consider the following issues.

Has a clear diagnosis of your problem been made? If a diagnosis cannot be made, then have other common conditions been excluded so that both you and your GP know that you are not missing out on appropriate conventional medical treatment?

If you have a chronic condition that is relatively stable then it may be reasonable to try a complementary medical approach, either to help your symptoms or to minimise the use of potentially damaging long-term conventional medicines. However, before you reduce your conventional medications, this must be discussed with your GP.

Your GP may regularly refer patients to a competent complementary therapist. If this is the case, your GP will be confident that the individual concerned is competent and safe.

Your GP may wish to refer you to another doctor practising some form of complementary medicine. This kind of referral should be exactly the same as a referral to any medically qualified specialist, because the person to whom your GP is referring you will be a registered medical practitioner.

As we have so little information about where complementary medicine may work best, it is quite reasonable to try a treatment (providing it is safe) for a limited period of time. You should agree with both your GP and your complementary practitioner, at the outset, when you would expect to see some beneficial effects.

Finding the right practitioner with so little information about which treatment works best in which condition is a difficult process. People seeking CAM often take advice from satisfied patients but, although this may help them find a competent complementary therapist, it is not always reliable. Sometimes individual therapy organisations can provide useful guidelines, but in general both you and your GP need to be assured that seeking complementary medical help is both appropriate and safe.

## HOW DO I KNOW MY THERAPIST IS COMPETENT?

If you are thinking of choosing a complementary therapist, then there are certain questions that you may like to ask. The answers will tell you if the practitioner is following the principles of good clinical practice but do not guarantee that they are competent.

**Do you think the practitioner is technically competent?** This usually means, is the practitioner a member of an appropriate organisation and does he or she have adequate training in the field in which he or she practises?

- Does the practitioner have professional indemnity? In other words, if the practitioner makes a mistake, is he or she insured?
- Does the practitioner have a code of ethics, are the data held about you legally protected and will he or she treat the information you give in a confidential manner?
- Is the practitioner part of an organisation that uses a process of self-regulation and that will remove members from their list if they are not behaving ethically?
- Is the practitioner aware of, and does he or she have a process of reporting, any adverse reaction to the treatment provided?

## HOW DO I KNOW MY THERAPIST IS COMPETENT? (contd)

**Could the practitioner advise you to change your conventional medical treatment without seeking the advice of your doctor?**

In general, it is a bad idea for one person treating you to suggest that you change treatments without communicating and informing the other people who are involved in your care. Ideally your GP should be talking with your complementary practitioner and vice versa.

**Can the proposed treatment be provided safely?**

For example, if you are seeing a herbalist, are you sure he or she is aware of the potential interactions between herbal medicine and any conventional medicines you may be taking?

**Will the complementary practitioner set guidelines with you, at the first appointment, for how he or she thinks the treatment should progress?**

Should you expect a response to treatment after three or four acupuncture sessions or would it be better to see what happens after eight or ten treatments? This helps to focus both your own mind and your practitioner's mind on whether the treatment is working.

At your first appointment, it would be helpful for you to take with you a clear list of your symptoms and problems; this can then be used to refer back to at a later stage because your symptoms may change during treatment.

The main organisations for you to contact are listed in Useful addresses, page 99.

In addition, both you and the practitioner need to develop a clear understanding of your objectives so that you get some improvement for a reasonable investment of time and money.

## Can I be referred on the NHS or will I need to pay privately?

There is some provision of CAM within the NHS. The homeopathic hospitals in London, Tunbridge Wells, Bristol and Glasgow have been part of the NHS since its inception in 1948. They offer a service that is largely homeopathic but also involves a comprehensive approach to a variety of CAM therapies, usually including acupuncture and manipulative medicine. Pain clinics and physiotherapy departments almost all offer acupuncture as part of their treatment regimens, and palliative care units dealing with patients who have terminal cancer often provide aromatherapy, reflexology and massage.

Complementary practitioners are increasingly forming part of the primary care team. In particular, during the whole process of GP fund-holding there were growing numbers of osteopaths, chiropractors and acupuncturists who were employed by general practices to offer a service to their patients. A recent BMA survey suggested that around 50 per cent of GPs referred patients for acupuncture and 15 per cent actually practised acupuncture on their own patients as part of their NHS commitment.

However, most complementary medicine practised in this country is within the private sector. Our research group has estimated, based on a questionnaire study, that approximately £4 million was spent on CAM consultations outside the NHS, in Southampton (population approximately 200,000) in 1996. The provision of CAM in the UK does not follow the clearly organised structure that exists within the NHS.

If you wish to seek some form of complementary medical treatment, you will probably need to pay privately. However, it is worth discussing it with your GP, as there may be an NHS referral route that is not widely publicised. You can usually obtain more information from the individual therapy organisations – for example, the Faculty of Homeopathy gives clear guidance to GPs on how they may refer patients through the NHS for homeopathy.

# Useful addresses

## General

### Association of Natural Medicine

19a Collingwood Road
Witham CM8 2DY
Tel: 01376 502762
Fax: 01376 502762
Email:
information@naturalmedicine.fsnet.co.uk
Website:
www.associationnaturalmedicine.co.uk

Promotes natural medicine through training in a wide range of complementary therapies. Offers support, training and registration for professional therapists. For information please send an SAE.

### Benefits Enquiry Line

Tel: 0800 882200
Website: dwp.gov.uk
Minicom: 0800 243355
N. Ireland: 0800 220674

Government agency giving information and advice on sickness and disability benefits for people with disabilities and their carers.

### British Complementary Medicine Association

PO Box 5122
Bournemouth BH8 0WG
Tel: 0845 345 5977
Fax: 0845 345 5978
Email: info@bcma.co.uk
Website: www.bcma.co.uk

Multi-therapy umbrella body representing organisations, clinics, colleges and independent schools, and acting as the voice of complementary medicine. Offers lists of qualified and insured practitioners of complementary medicine.

### British Holistic Medical Association

59 Lansdowne Place
Hove BN3 1FL
Tel: 01273 725951
Fax: 01273 725951
Email: bhma@bhma.org
Website: www.bhma.org

Promotes awareness of the holistic approach to health among practitioners and the general public through publications, self-help tapes, conferences and a network of local groups.

### Institute for Complementary Medicine

PO Box 194
London SE16 7QZ
Tel: 020 7237 5165
Fax: 020 7237 5175
Email: info@icmedicine.co.uk
Website: www.icmedicine.co.uk

Registered charity formed as umbrella for complementary medicine groups. Offers information and British register of accredited practitioners, and recommends approved training courses. An SAE requested with two first class stamps.

### National Institute for Clinical Excellence (NICE)

MidCity Place
71 High Holborn
London WC1V 6NA
Tel: 020 7067 5800
Fax: 020 7067 5801
Email: nice@nice.nhs.uk
Website: www.nice.org.uk

Provides guidance on treatments and care for people using the NHS in England and Wales. Patient information leaflets are available for each piece of guidance issued.

## Acupressure

### Shiatsu Society

Eastlands Court
St Peter's Road
Rugby CV21 3QP
Tel: 0845 130 4560
Fax: 01788 555052
Email: admin@shiatsu.org
Website: www.shiatsu.org

Represents all types and styles of shiatsu. Maintains a register of professional practitioners.

## Acupuncture

### Acupuncture Association of Chartered Physiotherapists

AACP Secretariat
Portcullis
Castle Street
Mere, Wilts BA12 6JE
Tel: 01747 861151
Fax: 01747 861171
Email: sec@aacp.uk.com
Website: www.aacp.uk.com

Non-profit-making association for chartered physiotherapists qualified in acupuncture treatment. For names of practitioners in your area please send an SAE.

### British Acupuncture Council

63 Jeddo Road
London W12 9HQ
Tel: 020 8735 0400
Fax: 020 8735 0404
Email: info@acupuncture.org.uk
Website: www.acupuncture.org.uk

Professional body offering lists of qualified acupuncture therapists in your area.

### British Medical Acupuncture Society

The Administrator
BMAS House
3 Winnington Court

Northwich WA8 1AQ
Tel: 01606 786782
Fax: 01606 786783
Email:
admin@medical-acupuncture.org.uk
Website:
www.medical-acupuncture.co.uk

Professional body offering training in acupuncture to doctors and a list of accredited practitioners in local areas.

## Aromatherapy

### Aromatherapy Consortium

PO Box 6522
Desborough
Kettering
Northants NN14 2YX
Tel: 0870 774 3477 (10am–2pm weekdays)
Fax: 0870 774 3477
Email:
info@aromatherapy-regulation.org.uk
Website:
aromatherapy-regulation.org.uk

Umbrella body representing aromatherapy associations that set national standards. Can provide details of local therapists, training and general information.

### International Federation of Aromatherapists

182 Chiswick High Road
London W4 1PP
Tel: 020 8742 2605
Fax: 020 8742 2606
Email: office@ifaroma.org
Website: www.ifaroma.org

Professional body that carries out research, sets standards and maintains register of training establishments which comply with their requirements. Can refer to qualified therapists in your area.

## Chiropractic

### British Chiropractic Association

Blagrave House
17 Blagrave Street
Reading RG1 1QB
Tel: 0118 950 5950
Fax: 0118 958 8946
Email: enquiries@chiropractic-uk.co.uk
Website: www.chiropractic-uk.co.uk

Professional body representing fully qualified chiropractors. Can refer to accredited practitioners in your area.

### General Chiropractic Council

44 Wicklow Street
London WC1X 9HL
Tel: 020 7713 5155
Fax: 020 7713 5844
Helpline: 0845 601 1796
Email: enquiries@gcc-uk.org
Website: www.gcc-uk.org

Professional body for chiropractors which can provide details of registered practitioners in your area.

## Healing

### Confederation of Healing Organisations

250 Chichester Road
North End
Portsmouth PO2 0AU
Tel: 02392 639275
Fax: 02392 713607
Email: tonyashendencho@ntlworld.com

Website: www.confederation-of-healing-organisations.org

Umbrella organisation for spiritual and other types of healing. Can refer to local healers.

### National Federation of Spiritual Healers

Old Manor Farm Studio
Church Street
Sunbury-on-Thames
Middlesex TW16 6RG
Tel: 0845 123 2777
Fax: 01932 779648
Healer referral line: 0845 123 2767
Email: office@nfsh.org.uk
Website: www.nfsh.org.uk

Trains and supports members to give healing to all who request it in private practice, healing centres and, when requested, in hospitals and hospices. Promotes research, coordinates distant healing and provides information and a national healer referral service.

## HERBAL MEDICINE

### British Herbal Medicine Association

1 Wickham Road
Boscombe
Bournemouth BH7 6JX
Tel: 01202 433691
Fax: 01202 417079
Email: secretary@bhma.info
Website: www.bhma.info

Offers information, encourages research and promotes high-quality standards. Advises members on legalities for importers, vets and advertisements, and defends the right of the public to choose herbal medicines and be able to obtain them safely.

### National Institute of Medical Herbalists (NIMH)

Elm House
54 Mary Arches Street
Exeter
Devon EX4 3BA
Tel: 01392 426022
Fax: 01392 498963
Email: nimh@ukexeter.freeserve.co.uk
Website: www.nimh.org.uk

Professional body representing qualified practising medical herbalists. Offers list of accredited medical herbalists. An SAE requested.

### Register of Chinese Herbal Medicine

Office 5
Ferndale Business Centre
1 Exeter Street
Norwich NR2 4QB
Tel: 01603 623994
Fax: 01603 667557
Email: herbmed@rchm.co.uk
Website: www.rchm.co.uk

Provides information to the public seeking properly qualified practitioners who are bound by code of ethics and insurance. Sets criteria for the practice and teaching of Chinese herbal medicine.

## Homeopathy

### British Homeopathic Association

Hahnemann House
29 Park Street West
Luton LU1 3BE
Tel: 0870 444 3950
Fax: 0870 444 3960
Email: info@trusthomeopathy.org
Website: www.trusthomeopathy.org

Professional body offering information about homeopathy and list of qualified practitioners.

### Society of Homeopaths

11 Brookfield
Duncan Close
Moulton Park
Northampton NN3 6WL
Tel: 0845 450 6611
Fax: 0845 450 6622
Email:info@homeopathy-soh.org
Website: www.homeopathy-soh.org

Professional body offering general information about homeopathy and list of accredited local therapists.

## Hypnotherapy

### Association of Qualified Curative Hypnotherapists

PO Box 9989
Birmingham B14 4WA
Tel: 0121 693 1223
Fax: 0121 693 1223
Email: info@aqch.org
Website: www.aqch.org

Organisation representing qualified curative hypnotherapists. Can recommend appropriate courses for training in this field.

### British Society of Medical and Dental Hypnosis

28 Dale Park Gardens
Cookridge
Leeds LS16 7PT
Tel: 07000 560309
Fax: 07000 560309
Email: nat.office@bsmdh.org
Website: www.bsmdh.com

Professional body offering training in hypnotherapy to doctors and dentists. Can provide list of accredited local medical and dental hypnotherapists.

### National Council for Hypnotherapy

PO Box 5779
Burton on the Wolds
Loughborough LE12 5ZF
Tel: 0800 952 0545
Email: admin@hypnotherapists.org.uk
Website: www.hypnotherapists.org.uk

Represents members, sets standards of practice and can refer to accredited training schools. Can put you in touch with a hypnotherapist in your area.

## Manipulative therapies

### British Institute of Musculoskeletal Medicine

34 The Avenue
Watford
Hertfordshire WD17 4AH
Tel: 01923 220999
Fax: 01923 249037
Email: info@bimm.org.uk
Website: www.bimm.org.uk

Charity promoting education and clinical research in the science of musculoskeletal medicine among the medical profession. Runs training courses and has a list of referral centres in the UK.

### Manipulation Association of Chartered Physiotherapists

14 Bedford Row
London WC1R 4ED
Tel: 020 7242 1941
Fax: 020 7306 6611
Email: enquiries@csp.org.uk
Website: www.csp.org.uk

An association of chartered physiotherapists with a particular clinical interest in manipulation.

## NUTRITIONAL MEDICINE

### Biolab Medical Unit

9 Weymouth Street
London W1W 6DB
Tel: 020 7636 5959
Fax: 020 7580 3910
Email: info@biolab.co.uk
Website: www.biolab.co.uk

Medical laboratory specialising in environmental medicine, measuring vitamins, minerals and other nutrients. Only accepts referrals from registered health professionals.

### British Association of Nutritional Therapists

27 Old Gloucester Street
London WC1N 3XX
Tel: 0870 606 1284
Fax: 0870 606 1284
Email: theadministrator@bant.org.uk
Website: www.bant.org.uk

Professional body promoting the highest standards of educational training and qualification in nutritional therapy. Has register of qualified members.

### British Dietetic Association

5th Floor, Charles House
148–149 Great Charles Street
Queensway
Birmingham B3 3HT
Tel: 0121 200 8080
Fax: 0121 200 8081
Email: info@bda.uk.com
Website: www.bda.uk.com

Professional association supporting dietitians; they can be contacted via hospitals or GP practices. For list of BDA-registered dietitians in private practice, please send an SAE.

### British Society for Allergy, Environmental and Nutritional Medicine

PO Box 7
Knighton
Powys LD7 1WT
Tel: 01547 550380
Fax: 01547 550339
Premium information line:
0906 302 0010
Email: info@bsaenm
Website: www.bsaenm.org

Represents health professionals working in this field and can refer to doctors in your area. Publishes information and lobbies for these topics to be included in the undergraduate curriculum.

### General Council and Register of Naturopaths

Goswell House
2 Goswell Road

Street BA16 0JG
Tel: 08707 456984
Fax: 08707 456985
Email: admin@naturopathy.org.uk
Website: www.naturopathy.org.uk

Establishes and maintains standards of education, inspects colleges and courses of naturopathy. Promotes investigations and research. Has register of people qualified to practise naturopathy.

## Osteopathy

### General Osteopathic Council

Osteopathy House
176 Tower Bridge Road
London SE1 3LU
Tel: 020 7357 6655
Fax: 020 7357 0011
Email: info@osteopathy.org.uk
Website: www.osteopathy.org.uk

Regulatory body that offers information about osteopathy to the public and lists of accredited osteopaths.

## Psychotherapy

### British Association of Psychotherapists

37 Mapesbury Road
London NW2 4HJ
Tel: 020 8452 9823
Fax: 020 8452 0310
Email: mail@bap-psychotherapy.org
Website: www.bap-psychotherapy.org

Training organisation representing psychotherapists. Can refer to qualified psychotherapists in your area.

### British Psychological Society

St Andrews House
48 Princess Road East
Leicester LE1 7DR
Tel: 0116 254 9568
Fax: 0116 247 0787
Email: enquiry@bps.org.uk
Website: www.bps.org.uk

Membership organisation representing psychologists and psychology in the UK. Has register of psychologists in your area.

### National Council of Psychotherapists

PO Box 6072
Nottingham NG6 9BW
Tel: 0845 230 6072
Fax: 0115 913 1382
Email: ncphq@ntl.com
Website:
www.natcouncilofpsychotherapists.org.uk

National association of psychotherapists, mainly in private practice, to whom the public may confidently refer.

## Reflexology

### Association of Reflexologists

27 Old Gloucester Street
London WC1N 3XX
Tel: 0870 567 3320
Fax: 01823 336646
Email: info@aor.org.uk
Website: www.aor.org.uk

Accreditation body offering lists of practitioners and training courses in reflexology.

### International Federation of Reflexologists

76–78 Edridge Road
Croydon
Surrey CR0 1EF
Tel: 020 8645 9134
Fax: 020 8649 9291
Email: ifr44@aol.com
Website: www.intfedreflexologists.org

Umbrella organisation representing reflexologists, offering information to the public and advice on suitable training.

### Scottish Institute of Reflexology

6/1 Mintoe Place
Hawick TD9 9JL
Tel: 01450 373135
Fax: 01450 373135
Email: info@scottishreflexology.org
Website: www.scottishreflexology.org.

Promotes, monitors and maintains the highest professional standards in reflexology among members and training establishments. Has register of accredited reflexologists who have public liability insurance.

## Yoga

### British Wheel of Yoga

25 Jermyn Street
Sleaford
Lincs NG34 7RU
Tel: 01529 306851
Fax: 01529 303233
Email: information@bwy.org.uk
Website: www.bwy.org.uk

Professional body offering lists of qualified yoga therapists. Also provides training courses in yoga.

### Yoga Biomedical Trust

Yoga Therapy Centre
90–92 Pentonville Street
London N1 9HS
Tel: 020 7689 3040
Fax: 020 7689 3048
Email: enquiries@yogatherapy.org
Website: www.yogatherapy.org

Charity developing and promoting research into yoga therapy, treating particular ailments and offering training of therapists. Centre offers on-site therapy.

### Yoga for Health Foundation

Ickwell Bury
Ickwell Green
Biggleswade
Beds SG18 9EF
Tel: 01767 627271
Fax: 01767 627266
Email:
admin@yogaforhealthfoundation.co.uk
Website:
www.yogaforhealthfoundation.co.uk

Offers teaching for remedial yoga at their own residential centre for people with health problems.

## The internet as a source of further information

After reading this book, you may feel that you would like further information on the subject. One source is the internet and there are a great many websites with useful information about medical disorders, related charities and support groups. Some websites, however, have unhelpful and inaccurate information. Many are sponsored by commercial organisations or raise revenue by advertising, but nevertheless aim to provide impartial and trustworthy health information. Others may be reputable but you should be aware that they may be biased in their recommendations. Remember that treatment advertised on international websites may not be available in the UK.

Unless you know the address of the specific website that you want to visit (for example familydoctor.co.uk), you may find the following guidelines helpful when searching the internet.

There are several different sorts of websites that you can use to look for information, the main ones being search engines, directories and portals.

### Search engines and directories

There are many search engines and directories that all use different algorithms (procedures for computation) to return different results when you do a search. Search engines use computer programs called spiders, which crawl the web on a daily basis to search individual pages within a site and then queue them ready for listing in their database.

Directories, however, consider a site as a whole and use the description and information that was provided with the site when it was submitted to the directory to decide whether a site matches the searcher's needs. For both there is little or no selection in terms of quality of information, although engines and directories do try to impose rules about decency and content. Popular search engines in the UK include:

google.co.uk
aol.co.uk
msn.co.uk
lycos.co.uk
hotbot.co.uk
overture.com
ask.co.uk
espotting.com
looksmart.co.uk
alltheweb.com
uk.altavista.com

The two biggest directories are:

yahoo.com (yahoo.co.uk allows you to search UK sites only)
dmoz.org

### Portals

Portals are doorways to the internet that provide links to useful sites, news and other services, and may also provide search engine services (such as msn.co.uk). Many portals charge for putting their clients' sites high up in your list of search results. The quality of the websites listed depends on the selection criteria used in compiling the portal, although portals focused on a specific group, such as medical information portals, may have more rigorous inclusion criteria than other searchable websites. Examples of medical portals can be found at:

nhsdirect.nhs.uk
patient.co.uk

Links to many British medical charities will be found at the Association of Medical Research Charities (www.amrc.org.uk) and Charity Choice (www.charitychoice.co.uk).

### Search phrases

Be specific when entering a search phrase. Searching for information on 'cancer' could give astrological information as well as medical: 'lung cancer' would be a better choice. Either use the engine's advanced search feature and ask for the exact phrase, or put the phrase in quotes – 'lung cancer' – as this will link the words. Adding 'uk' to your search phrase will bring up mainly British websites, so a good search would be 'lung cancer' uk (don't include uk within the quotes).

Always remember that the internet is international and unregulated. Although it holds a wealth of invaluable information, individual websites may be biased, out of date or just plain wrong. Family Doctor Publications accepts no responsibility for the content of links published in their series.

# Index